MANAGING THE HEAVY METALS ON THE LAND

POLLUTION ENGINEERING AND TECHNOLOGY

A Series of Reference Books and Textbooks

EDITORS

1. Energy from Solid Wastes, *Paul N. Cheremisinoff and Angelo C. Morresi*
2. Air Pollution Control and Design Handbook (in two parts), *edited by Paul N. Cheremisinoff and Richard A. Young*
3. Wastewater Renovation and Reuse, *edited by Frank M. D'Itri*
4. Water and Wastewater Treatment: Calculations for Chemical and Physical Processes, *Michael J. Humenick, Jr.*
5. Biofouling Control Procedures, *edited by Loren D. Jensen*
6. Managing the Heavy Metals on the Land, *G. W. Leeper*

Additional volumes in preparation

MANAGING THE HEAVY METALS ON THE LAND

G. W. Leeper

Emeritus Professor of Agricultural Chemistry
University of Melbourne, Australia

Consultant to Sheaffer & Roland, Inc.
Chicago, Illinois

1978

MARCEL DEKKER, INC. New York and Basel

Library of Congress Cataloging in Publication Data

Leeper, Geoffrey Winthrop.
Managing the heavy metals on the land.

(Pollution engineering and technology; v. 6)
Bibliography: p.
Includes index.
1. Soil pollution. 2. Sewage irrigation.
3. Plants, Effect of heavy metals on. I. Title.
II. Series.
TD879.H4L43 631.7 77-20934
ISBN 0-8247-6661-X

MARCEL DEKKER, INC.

270 Madison Avenue, New York, New York 10016

Current printing (last digit):
10 9 8 7 6 5 4 3 2 1

PRINTED IN THE UNITED STATES OF AMERICA

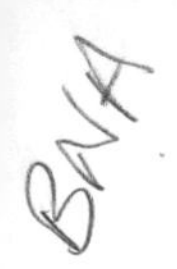

CONTENTS

PREFACE v

SUMMARY FOR THE GENERAL READER vii

1. INTRODUCTION 1

2. FORMS OF HEAVY METALS 5

2.1 The Center of Soil Chemistry 5

2.2 General Statements about Heavy Metals 10

2.3 The Reactions of Heavy Metals with Sludge and Soil 11

2.4 The Mechanisms of Removal of Individual Heavy Metals 26

2.5 Estimates of Mobile Heavy Metals 35

2.6 Heavy Metals in Nature 39

3. RELATIONS OF PLANTS TO THE HEAVY METALS 45

3.1 Differences among Plants 46

3.2 Antagonism 48

3.3 Information from Simplified Systems 49

3.4 Uptake and Tolerance of Zinc 52

3.5 Uptake and Tolerance of Copper 54

3.6 Uptake and Tolerance of Cadmium 54

3.7 Uptake and Tolerance of Nickel 59

3.8 Uptake and Tolerance of Lead 60

4. CROPPING WITH SEWAGE WASTES CONTAINING HEAVY METALS 61

4.1 Nature of Sewage Sludge 61

4.2 Cropping with Sewage and Sludge Applied at High Rates 68

4.3 Cropping with Sludge Applied at Low Rates; Sludge Considered as Source of Phosphate 88

4.4 Heavy Metals in Irrigation Water from Secondary Treatment 90

4.5 Accumulation of Metals in Food Crops 91

4.6 Management 93

5. TWO FUTURE INQUIRIES 105

5.1 Practice and Theory 105

REFERENCES 107

REVIEWS AND SOURCES 115

INDEX OF SYSTEMATIC NAMES 117

INDEX 119

PREFACE

This book has been written in order to explain and summarize the chemical and biological issues that arise when the products of a sewage system containing heavy metals are applied to agricultural land. It is above all an attempt to clarify a field which will be much debated in the next few years and in which some strong feelings exist, some of which might dissipate if the subject were better understood.

The main body of the book uses theoretical concepts and terms which, while familiar to a student of physical chemistry, are strange to many readers who wish to inform themselves on the central issues at stake. (This is a perpetual problem with the world of soil, in which one can travel only a small way before facing such concepts.) For the benefit of the more general reader, a summary chapter has been written which precedes the main book and can be read independently.

My involvement in the subject began with my work on the trace elements in plant nutrition, both in theory and experiment, during my career at the University of Melbourne. After retiring from the chair of Agricultural Chemistry at that university I wrote a book, Six Trace Elements in Soils, in which six heavy metals were discussed, with special regard to how soils may hold these back from plants in situations where they are vitally needed. I was later invited to summarize the opposite side, namely how soils may hold back heavy metals from plants in situations where they are in excess and so liable to do damage. This summary was issued in 1973 as a typescript by the U.S.A. Corps of Engineers as Contract DACW-73-73-CW26. The present book includes most of that summary. It has been much expanded to include, in particular, discussions of the composition of sludges and experimental accounts of the impact of heavy metals in sewage applied in agriculture in several industrial countries. It was written while I was acting as consultant for Bauer, Sheaffer and Lear, Inc. of Chicago.

Work on many sides of this subject has expanded greatly since my first summary was made in 1972. This is especially illustrated by the holding of an international conference on Heavy Metals in the Environment in Toronto in October 1975, in which about sixty papers fell within the area of this book. Some of these papers point towards answers to some of the questions raised in the following pages. But the aim throughout this book has been to outline and explain, not to be bibliographic.

Any reader who expects to find here ready answers in numerical terms should be warned that, while a few questions may be answered simply, for the most part exact answers cannot be given since the most vexed questions involve forecasts of slow changes in the soil projected five or ten years ahead. Rather I hope that if the principles here discussed are more widely understood, decisions may be made more intelligently.

Any conclusions or opinions that are expressed herein are my own. But any book is something of a collective effort, to which the ideas and criticisms of various readers and other colleagues have contributed. While I am grateful to many colleagues, I would like to acknowledge in particular the help of Dr. R. L. Chaney, Dr. L. H. P. Jones, Dr. N. C. Uren, and Mr. John Lear; and especially Dr. J. R. Sheaffer, to whose enthusiasm the creation of this book is due. I would like also to thank Lee Cochran who typed many drafts of the book.

G. W. Leeper

SUMMARY
FOR THE GENERAL READER

Soil is almost all insoluble, otherwise it would not be there. For our present purpose we may ignore the few parts per hundred of living things and their residues; they are important in their cycling of the essential elements of life — nitrogen, phosphorus, and the rest — but they make up only a small part of the total. We are here concerned with the 90 percent, or commonly the 95 percent, that makes up the inorganic or mineral skeleton, the skeleton which has its own use in containing pores of all sizes, some small enough to hold water as a reserve for plants, some large enough to drain off water soon after rain and so to allow air to enter from above.

The dominant mineral of the world's soils is quartz — silica, SiO_2 , the main component of sand and silt. It is so inert that it is commonly used experimentally as the solid medium for growing plants in nutrient culture. The plants are given their necessary dozen elements in aqueous solution, and the grains of silica form the bed for the roots. Minute amounts dissolve, and silica enters into all the world's plants as a neutral and harmless molecule.

But when we turn to the next most plentiful elements after silicon and oxygen, namely aluminum and iron, we already find an introduction to what will be our main theme on the heavy metals. Aluminum is a major element in the crystalline silicates of the igneous rocks, and through them in the weathered clays that characterize the world's soils; kaolinite, the most familiar of the clays, is 21 percent aluminum. This element, universally present in soils, is toxic to most of our cultivated crops. True, many plants growing wild in nature and some species and some varieties of cultivated crops take up large amounts of aluminum without harm, but most crops can tolerate only very small amounts. The reason for this contrast is that aluminum dissolves only in an acid environment; in the common range of cultivated soils, through mildly acid to neutral to calcareous, the amounts in solution are negligible. Farmers have long since found that some soils must be treated with lime in order to reduce their acidity; in more modern terms, to keep the pH above (say) 5.5.* One reason for doing this is to keep the amounts of soluble aluminum below the danger point. So we have our first example of farming safely in spite of the apparent danger in the soil. We could expand our example further, since man may decide in some regions to live with the problem and to grow only tolerant crops. The potato has long been found to tolerate, even to prefer, acid soils, and varieties of wheat have been developed to tolerate solúble aluminum. Some plants that have developed a mechanism for living healthily on acid soils may come to require acidity, and many gardeners know the species which must on no account be limed, of which perhaps the rhododendron is best known.

Iron was mentioned above as one of the plentiful elements in soils. It is like aluminum in its chemistry, only more so; it is removed from solution so easily that even at a pH of 4, which is as low as occurs in a natural soil, the amounts in solution are minute. The perpetual problem with iron in soil is how a plant succeeds in extracting its necessary supply of 100 grams from an acre that contains 10 tons of iron within reach of the roots. This is a problem to which there is no generally agreed answer; not only is it a theoretical problem, but in many regions of the world a severely practical one, since the cultivated plant may languish for lack of

---

*The pH scale runs from highly acidic (zero or even negative) through neutral to highly alkaline (14 or more). The pHs of the great majority of the world's soils lie between 4.5 and 9.5. The range from 6.5 to 7.5 is often considered as neutral; going up from this range one passes from slightly to strongly alkaline, and going down one passes from slightly to strongly acidic.

the iron surrounding it, one hundred-thousandth of which would satisfy its needs. It is particularly the acid-loving species referred to in the preceding paragraph that are thus poorly equipped for digging out their necessary quota of iron.

So much for the main constituents of mineral soil. Next let us consider two metals which while minor are substantial, namely titanium and manganese. Titanium oxide, TiO_2, often occurs to the extent of 1 percent in soils. It is so insoluble, in both acid, neutral, and alkaline soils, that it is suitably ignored when nutrition or toxicity is under discussion. But manganese has a more varied chemistry. Briefly expressed, it may be insoluble as MnO_2 in well-aerated neutral and alkaline soils, and may be soluble as the manganous ion both in well-drained acidic soils and in waterlogged neutral as well as acidic soils. Such a common reserve as 300 parts per million (ppm) of soil may liberate toxic amounts of manganese to solution when a soil is either acidified or waterlogged, and many examples could be quoted of cultivated crops being so damaged. But most areas containing such reserves are not so mishandled, and they are used successfully over generations. As with aluminum, different species and local strains of crops vary greatly in their tolerance of manganese. Like iron and unlike aluminum, manganese is needed in small amounts by all plants, and a crop may fail for lack of available manganese on some neutral s soils which contain some thousands-fold of its needs.

In these introductory paragraphs, the natural occurrence of two heavy metals in soils, iron and manganese, has been discussed; perhaps titanium is too light to qualify as a third. Before turning to the core of our subject, namely the heavy metals that are added to soils through sewage wastes, one should discuss another element that is plentiful in soils, namely barium, which is often quoted as occurring as one part per thousand. We will later be concerned with the possible damage of heavy metals to crops, but there is little or no information about such damage by barium in nature. Its interest is different; namely, that the element may accumulate in edible parts of plants in such large amounts as to damage or kill an animal or human consumer. Barium is a common rat poison and is toxic to humans, three-quarters of a gram being quoted as a lethal dose. Most of our edible crops contain only a few parts of barium per million, and are perfectly safe. The brazil nut, however, collects barium and has been reported as containing 0.5 percent (5,000 ppm) in the edible part. The existence of this exceptional collector emphasizes the fact that man has lived for a million years unharmed with this deadly element in his soils.

After this introduction we may consider the heavy metals that may be added to soils with sewage wastes both solid and liquid. While more than half the elements known to man may be called "heavy metals," metallic like iron and heavy like iron, no more than 12 of these call for discussion here, namely those that are used and discharged by industrial communities in such amounts as to double or multiply the amounts normally present in soil. The 12, in alphabetical order, are cadmium, chromium, cobalt, copper, iron, lead, manganese, mercury, molybdenum, nickel, tin, and zinc.* Of these 12, detailed attention is commonly confined to four, as will be seen.

One must emphasize the fact that all these metals occur in small amounts in all soils, whether contaminated or not. Mankind has lived in their company over past ages — and in fact has always needed minute amounts of many of them for health, which shows that they must always have been widely distributed. The problem is nothing like that of adding a new creation like, say, DDT; it is one of increasing something already there. Soils and plants have mechanisms that make the original amounts innocuous; is there some point at which these saving mechanisms become inefficient?

To return to our detailed list: first, the added iron and manganese do not constitute a problem, since both elements are already present in much larger amounts in the soil than are added in

* Other elements that may also be added to soils through sewage include boron, arsenic, and selenium. These are not metals, and besides their chemical behavior in soils differs greatly from that of zinc and its associates, so they are excluded from this discussion. Boron is the only element of those here discussed on which there is much printed information on excess amounts in soils and irrigation waters and the tolerance of many economic crops.

wastes. If the added manganese were to present a problem by becoming soluble, then so would the native manganese under the same conditions. It is sensible, therefore, to confine discussion to what we might call the "foreign" metals — that is, to the remaining 10.

Second, some of these added metals are in a form, or are converted into a form, in which they remain immobile, neither entering into solution nor into a biological cycle. This is clearly so with chromium, which forms the insoluble oxide Cr_2O_3. Lead and mercury added to soil have likewise shown no trace of increasing in plant uptake or of entering into drainage. The statement that mercury rates no more than this mention may surprise a reader who knows of the harm done to aquatic life by discharges of mercury into lakes and estuaries. But these are quite different situations from soil. In water, mercury may be carried on very fine suspended particles and may even be dissolved off these particles on meeting the salt sea. But applied in sludges to soil, it is strongly precipitated on the spot so is filtered out, and is not taken up at all by roots, so that unlike its toxic relative cadmium it does not enter the food chain. Lead too may endanger life through aerial contamination, but not by entering the edible parts of plants by way of the soil. Tin (of which less is known in soil chemistry than of lead) similarly shows no evidence of entering into circulation. So these four may be regarded as no different from titanium in their performance in soils. We may also agree to omit cobalt from discussion, since while it is as toxic as nickel, it is present in wastes in far lower amounts.

Molybdenum has been included in this first full list, but it does not call for more than a passing mention. A few soils are known in which molybdenum enters pasture plants in amounts toxic for livestock, but none are known in which molybdenum from sewage wastes has led to any such toxicity, and the amounts so added are likely to remain too small for concern.

There remain zinc, copper, nickel, and cadmium, all of which must be considered individually: zinc, copper, and nickel, because all are on record as having damaged certain crops when applied with sewage sludge; and cadmium, because it is on record as having accumulated in some plants to levels dangerous to the consumer. Whether added in solution or in sludge, all these metals are bound strongly by soil and remain there permanently, with only minute proportions reaching the drainage system. (This statement is made about normal soil, not about sands.) At the same time, in spite of their strong binding, they are taken up by roots and thence into the tops, in amounts greater than in untreated soils. These amounts may be excessive; the result depends on the crop and the soil as well as on the composition of the sludge or solution. Weight for weight, nickel is much more toxic than zinc; on the other hand, it is commonly present in much lower amounts in sludges.

The amounts concerned are exemplified by a sludge containing 3,000 ppm of zinc; an application of 40 tons/acre of such sludge would add 1/8 ton of zinc or 120 ppm in the surface soil compared with the common natural figure of one-half as much. (Zinc is commonly used in these illustrations because it is the dominant "foreign metal" in sludge.)

The three interacting entities — plant, soil, and sludge — may be considered in order. First, different species of plants differ greatly in their uptake of each metal, and not only do species differ but so do varieties, so that one might find a tolerant strain of a generally sensitive species. Most of the common grasses and grain crops are tolerant of these heavy metals, while the leafy vegetables, especially the beets, are easily damaged.

Second, soils differ in two ways, first in colloid content (which we may define as material less than one-fifth a micrometer in diameter, 0.0002 millimeter) and second in pH. The full mechanism by which they bind heavy metals is not well known and is controversial, but at least this is agreed. The organic colloid ("humus") may be five times as effective as the same percentage of clay (the inorganic colloid). But the effect depends on pH, with a sharp increase in binding from 6 upwards. Thus acidic soils involve far more risk of damage than do those close to neutrality.

Third, sludge itself inactivates the heavy metals which it incorporates, in two ways. First, by virtue of its own organic composition; second, by its content of inorganic phosphorus, namely 2 or 3 percent of dry weight, to quote a common value in the United States. This phosphate antagonizes the heavy metals inside the plant, rather than within the soil.

Information on the heavy application of heavy metals with sewage wastes may come from continuous usage over many years or from a single application at a heavy rate. The question of whether these two treatments give similar or contrasting results leads us into the controversy just referred to — namely, what is the binding mechanism?

In short, soil is a universal precipitating agent by virtue of its colloidal constituents. The form into which a heavy metal is immediately bound may be loose enough to allow a substantial proportion to move a little and to enter and damage plants. But in the days or months after its addition to soil it is likely to rearrange into ever more stable and less soluble forms. While some exact statements may be made about the ultimate, most stable and least soluble forms, such statements do not help us; our problem is at what rate the rearranging happens, and here no answer is given by theory, and conflicting answers may be given in practice. It has long been known that light applications of zinc (2 or 3 pounds/acre) disappear from circulation within a few days, but this is not true of 200 or 300 pounds/acre. When zinc has been added to soil with sludge, two opposing effects follow in the next few years: on the one hand, the organic components of the sludge, which had been helping to bind it, are destroyed by microbial oxidation; on the other, its compounds with other components of the soil are rearranging themselves towards lower solubility. One of the debatable issues in this complex affair is how much credit to give to the soil for its protection and how much to sludge. The sludge may be very efficient while it lasts, but it may oxidize away so that half has disappeared in 3 or 4 years — that is, its protecting power is halved.

In general, zinc and cadmium remain more soluble for longer in soils than do copper and nickel, so call for more serious attention when sludge is added.

In all such experiences, whether practical as in city sewage farms, or partly or wholly experimental, the major cases of direct damage by heavy metals added in sewage or sludge have been with vegetable crops, whether by zinc, copper, or nickel. Indirect damage by the antagonism of zinc against manganese or (probably) against copper has been noted, but such antagonisms are easily dealt with in the field. Liming the soil has often succeeded in overcoming the direct damage.

Formulas have been proposed for calculating the safe limits of addition of heavy metals when sensitive crops are to be grown. One such, as set out by the Environmental Protection Agency of the United States in PL 92:500, is illustrated and expanded in Table I. The two properties of the soil analyzed are pH and cation exchange capacity (c.e.c.) which is a routine determination measuring the holding power of a soil.

The accompanying table shows the tolerable loadings of zinc in three kinds of soil: first, an ordinary one; second, one with higher clay content and therefore especially favorable for the present purpose; third, a sand. The central figure for each soil, namely pH 6.5, gives the suggested upper limit set by E.P.A. The doubling or halving for an increase or decrease, respectively, of half a unit of pH are my own suggestions, which are given some theoretical and practical backing in the book. All figures have been rounded off so as to avoid any pretence to accuracy. The reader must be reminded that to lower the pH by half a unit means, by definition, to multiply the acidity by 3.16.

Two properties here tabulated are partly under the control of the farmer, namely pH and c.e.c. The pH can be raised by the traditional practice of liming. The c.e.c. is mostly determined naturally by the proportions of sand and clay in the soil, but it can be increased by increasing the organic content, at the rate of 2 to 4 for each 1 percent organic matter. Again, this is a matter of farming practice.

The table has over-simplified the situation in one important respect. Since zinc is usually the major heavy metal in sludge, it is a good starting point for discussion. But some sludges contain also relatively substantial amounts of copper and nickel. Formulas have been devised for allowing for the added risk of these metals, which are more toxic to plants than zinc. These formulas rely on arbitrary figures for weighting the copper and nickel (as discussed in the book). They will clearly result in a lower figure of tolerance than is given in the table. But practical demonstrations are quoted

TABLE I

Suggested Safe Limits of Zinc for Sensitive Crops in Three Kinds of Soil Managed at Three pH Levels

Texture of soil	Cation exchange capacity (c.e.c.)	pH	Percentage of c.e.c. safely occupied with zinc	Added zinc pound/acre -7 inch (safe level)	Equiv. tons sludge at 3,000 ppm zinc	Years of irrigation, zinc at 1 ppm 60 inch annually
Average	15	6.0	5	490	85	35
		6.5	10	980	165	65
		7.0	20	1,960	330	135
Clayey	30	6.0	5	980	165	65
		6.5	10	1,960	330	135
		7.0	20	3,920	655	265
Sand	3	6.0	5	100	17	7
		6.5	10	200	33	14
		7.0	20	390	65	27

in the following pages where the loadings given by these formulas have been much exceeded without any sign of damage to major crops (which are more resistant than are some of the leafy vegetables) and without any pollution of drainage water.

Cadmium calls for special consideration, as an element that some crops will accumulate without obvious damage to themselves but in amounts that are toxic to a consumer. Among the other elements of our discussion only molybdenum behaves like this (though barium in nature provides a striking example, as we have seen). Copper could conceivably accumulate to concentrations damaging to grazing ruminants, but this does not seem to happen with sewage treatments, and on the sewage farm of Melbourne, Australia, where over a hundred pounds of copper have accumulated per acre, the grazing cattle are slightly deficient in copper.

There is as yet no agreement on the limits of safety for cadmium in food, either for short-lived livestock or for human beings and long-lived animals in general (as cadmium accumulates in animal organs with age). The problem is complicated by the fact that other elements antagonize it within animals, and further by doubt on the accuracy of some of the published figures. Many plant analyses in nature give cadmium contents of about half a part per million of dry matter; yet this is the figure which is proposed by some workers as the upper tolerable limit for human food.

Cadmium is present in many city sludges to the order of 100 ppm of dry weight. Adding 10 tons of this to an acre-7 inches of soil would incorporate 1 ppm total cadmium in the soil, which is 3 to 10 times as much as is held by an average soil. Crops grown with sludges containing cadmium have been found to contain 10 to 20 ppm in their leaves. Perhaps the only sure way to keep the cadmium out of food coming from such treated land is to grow only grain crops which exclude cadmium from the grain (as most of them do) and to return the leaves to the soil.

The reader may have concluded that one's first object should be to reduce the amount of heavy metal in sludges, and that some of the contents quoted in the following pages are inexcusably high.

This is not under dispute. However, this book is concerned with the impact of heavy metals on soils — whether added as sewage sludge or effluent, or otherwise as in composts in urban gardens — and some examples are usefully drawn from sludges of very high metallic content, which have been outdated for some years. One may expect a further improvement and reduction in these contents in years to come. But the core of the problem will remain in an industrial society since copper and zinc, in particular, are so widely used domestically as well as industrially.

Sewage or sludge may be applied to land simply as a way of disposing of a nuisance. Thought of in this way, one may favorably compare the addition of the accompanying heavy metal to a soil, from which it does not move further, with the two alternative disposals, namely to the air (by incineration) or to water, both of which increase the general environmental level of a noxious metal. But application to the land does much more than dispose of a nuisance, since it simultaneously allows some of the major nutrients to be recovered, and while initially it may be thought of as providing revenue for a municipal farm, it can confer agricultural benefit on a wider scale. One aim may be to use up the organic nitrogen and so to recycle the nitrogen in growing crops. In such a case the total amounts applied are heavy, and the amounts of heavy metal simultaneously applied are themselves heavy. But in all such cases the amount of phosphorus applied is enormous, being many times as much as would be needed for the maximum yield of a crop. From this line of thought comes the proposal to recycle, not nitrogen but phosphorus, so to limit the application of sewage sludge to the amount of phosphate required for one cropping year. This involves reducing the addition of heavy metal to about one-fiftieth or one-hundredth of the amount previously discussed — or otherwise expressed, spreading it over fifty or one hundred times the area. This greatly postpones any future day of reckoning. The heavy metals will still accumulate in the surface soil, but only zinc and cadmium are likely to remain active enough in soil over the decades to enter into food chains, and of these only cadmium is a serious hazard. Now that its noxiousness is recognized one may expect that its addition to sludges will be steadily reduced; and more will be learned about the crops and varieties that exclude it from their edible parts.

The other addition of heavy metal to consider is as liquid effluent, which recycles nutrients and often supplies water in excess of the plants' needs. The heavy metal content may be 0.5 ppm of copper and nickel and 1 ppm of zinc; the reported figures for cadmium are too low to attach meaning to. These figures exaggerate the danger, since contents of heavy metals in effluents are usually well below these figures and may be expected to decrease further in the coming years. But if we accept them, reference to the table shows that such amounts of zinc added through irrigation water to a sandy soil, with a c.e.c. no more than 3 m.e. per 100 gram, would be too great, and the metal might both enter crops in damaging amounts, and also pass without hindrance through the soil into drainage.

The last paragraph brings us back to the themes of caution and uncertainty that surround the subject. It is no light matter to decide to multiply the naturally occurring burdens of heavy metals in soils by a factor of 3 to 5. Yet most soils can carry such burdens without our incurring any more serious penalty than the need for occasionally liming the soil to near the neutral point.

MANAGING THE HEAVY METALS ON THE LAND

CHAPTER 1

INTRODUCTION

The breadth and extent of interest in possible excesses of heavy metals in agricultural soils is new, and is directly related to the renewed interest in applying sewage wastes, including both sludge and treated effluent, to the land. However, there has long been some interest in such excesses. Some trace elements now recognized as essential in small amounts were first regarded as only obnoxious in larger amounts, notably boron, manganese, and selenium. Among other natural excesses, that of nickel on serpentine soils has often aroused interest. More interest was taken in the accumulation of the pesticide lead arsenate, which added two toxic elements, and of the fungicidal Bordeaux mixture, which added copper — a less severe poison than lead or arsenic, but still a poison. It was recognized that all these elements once added were with us permanently. While most soils could fix lead and arsenate (at least in the amounts then applied) in forms harmless to plants, some were affected by the copper so that they would not grow crops unless limed.

While the theme of possible excess will dominate the book, it should be made clear from the start that the elements under discussion here occur in small amounts in all soils, whether contaminated or not, and that man has always lived with them unharmed (apart from the few above-named natural excesses). The issue to which we shall return is, how well can man live with twice as much, or twice as much again, as was there originally.

The return of human wastes to the land is as old as settled agriculture. In this way the valuable nutrient elements — nitrogen and phosphorus in particular, but other major and minor nutrients besides — are used for raising succeeding crops and so are kept in circulation. When the same principle is applied to a modern urban sewage system, water also may be thus reclaimed for reuse. There has been increasing interest in the United States of America in the 1970's for so recycling the wastes of large cities, using the solid sludge as a fertilizer and physical amendment, and the liquid effluent for irrigation as well as a fertilizer. This involves several engineering and hygienic problems and some chemical problems which are not our concern here (such as possible excess of ammonium or nitrate or other soluble salts). Only one serious trouble remains; sewage comes from the houses and factories of the industrial age, so both sludge and effluent, to very different degrees as will be seen, carry a burden of heavy metals far greater than that introduced in normal diet. This book discusses the nature and severity of this burden, which carries two risks, one of direct damage to crops, the other of excessive uptake causing damage to the consumer. These will bc discussed sometimes together, sometimes separately.

Two further uses of sewage wastes may be mentioned here, though they are not discussed in the book; namely, in forestry and in reclaiming strip-mined areas. Where a forest area is sprayed with effluent there is a double intention, to increase growth and to produce a drinkable water in the streams after soil and trees have played their part; since human nutrition is not directly concerned, the heavy metals added to the land are easily ignored. For reclaiming strip-mined areas, sludge is often applied to start plants in a new soil and protect them against heavy metal in the subsoil, so the presence of a little more heavy metal in the sludge is of little account.

The meaning of the term "heavy metal" depends on the context. In this book it will largely coincide with the heavy metals of industry, since in a less industrial age the problem would not exist; copper and zinc in particular come from domestic sources as well as from factories. Most of the discussion will be confined to a few of those named, but the full list comprises cadmium (Cd), chromium (Cr), cobalt (Co), copper (Cu), iron (Fe), lead (Pb), manganese (Mn), mercury (Hg), molybdenum (Mo), nickel (Ni), tin (Sn), and zinc (Zn). Boron and arsenic, two other elements that are sometimes present in high amounts in sewage, are not metals as defined by chemists, and the chemistry of each of them is distinct enough to warrant their exclusion here. Selenium, another non-metallic element, is unlikely to be present in important amounts.

The word "foreign" will be used below for all those in the above list except Fe and Mn. In a strictly literal use of the word, no element is foreign to soils since traces of everything are in water and air as well as in rock. But in a less extreme use the word is apt. Going back to the original igneous rocks, many metals are segregated in ores when the magmas crystallize. Only small proportions of some of the heavy metals remain in the bulk of the magma and eventually crystallize out in common minerals like augite as impurities, substitutes for commoner elements by the accident of having the same size; and it is from these impurities that we may picture the essential trace elements Co and Cu and Mo and Zn entering universally into soils and waters. Their normal concentrations in soils are low, so if one brings in as much as five times that amount in sludge a new situation arises which may or may not have serious biological results. It is in this sense that the heavy metals are called foreign, except for Fe and Mn of which Fe normally exceeds 1% of the soil and Mn often reaches 0.05%, as contrasted with Mo with 0.0002% or 2 ppm.

The first 12 elements making up the inorganic matter of soils are silicon (Si), aluminum (Al), iron (Fe), oxygen (O), hydrogen (H), manganese (Mn), titanium (Ti), barium (Ba), calcium (Ca), magnesium (Mg), potassium (K), sodium (Na). These most plentiful elements already include two that are often toxic to plants at low pH (Al, Mn) and one (Ba) that is highly toxic to animals. We rely on mechanisms within the soil and the plant for keeping these elements circulating only in appropriately low amounts; and these mechanisms have been naturally so efficient for Ba that few people know that this element, three quarters of a gram of which can kill a man, is among the twelve most plentiful in soils.

We have here an introduction to our main theme. What are the amounts of active heavy metals in soils that lead to troubles in plants or in their consumers, whether human beings or farm livestock? By what mechanisms are plants and animals protected? An understanding of these mechanisms is needed in deciding on the right agricultural management.

The reader will perceive that some of the subject is obscure and controversial, including such an important piece of chemistry as the reaction between zinc and organic matter; and that some answers are speculative. But a background of theory and experiment such as discussed here is important for making decisions in the years ahead.

It has to be assumed in discussing chemical topics that the reader is familiar with the ideas of physical chemistry covered by terms such as colloid, metastable, pH, millimolar and micromolar, oxidation and reduction. The "Summary for the General Reader," however, has been written to meet the needs of a reader who has not this familiarity. All units other than in that chapter are metric, including the ton.

CHAPTER 2

FORMS OF HEAVY METALS

2.1 THE CENTER OF SOIL CHEMISTRY

The center of soil chemistry so far as plants are concerned is the question, What are the forms and reactions of each of the elements that may be taken up by plants? For every such element there is a cycle through soil, through plant, through animal, back to soil, with perhaps changes in valence, changes between ionic and covalent state, and changes in neighbors. The best known such cycle, that of nitrogen, is most complex. Silicon, at the other extreme, moves as silicic acid through soil into plant and may complete a cycle in this molecular form or may change its state of aggregation to plant opal and no more. Our heavy metals are intermediate between these two; they mostly keep to the one valence but may vary greatly in their solubility during their sojourn within the soil, and this is our main interest.

The subject may well be introduced with the element phosphorus (P), which always is present in the soil as phosphate (PO_4). Most of the world's soils are deficient in P; an early step in developing agriculture in industrial countries has been to add P fertilizer. It is commonly observed that more P must be added in each successive year for a long time after breaking new land. Only a minor part of the added P is recovered in the harvest; most of it remains in the surface soil where it was placed, and the value of each lot of this residual P diminishes year by year. Yet after many years of addition, perhaps 50, the greed of the precipitating agents, whether aluminum or iron or calcium, is largely satisfied, and the supply of the soluble P becomes satisfactory, even if a small supplement may still be needed for a maximum harvest. This diminution in value of applied P has been called "reversion." This curious term was first used for phosphate when it was observed that much of the applied P was not taken up by the crop, and that what remained of a previous year's application of P was much less than a current application, so it was said that the P had reverted to its original form, namely rock phosphate. While this idea is incorrect, the term "reversion" is still useful for the change of any residual fertilizer into a second-class or third-class form.

We say "second-class" or "third-class." An element that has precipitated in the soil may become steadily less available with time. The first precipitate, whatever it may be, is poorly crystalline and has a high specific surface. As the weeks and years pass it reorganizes and becomes more regular, with a lower specific surface. But the third-class form is not altogether inert, and it is useful to think of our total supply to solution as compounded in the following numerical way.

Suppose that an element can be classified into three forms, A, B, and C, which may be called first-class, second-class, and third-class. They liberate their supply of the element into solution at the respective rates of 50%, 5%, and 0.1% per annum (of course there is a continuous range from the most to the least soluble, but that does not upset this argument). Suppose further, for the sake of simplicity, that the soil is in equilibrium with plants, which use

TABLE 2.1

Classes of Element and Rates of Liberation

Class of supply	Total, kg/ha	Rate of liberation, %	Delivery kg/ha per annum
A	20	50	10
B	100	5	5
C	1,000	0.1	1

the soluble supply as fast as it is liberated and restore it to the soil when they die. Then we construct Table 2.1 as shown opposite.

This total delivery of 16 kg will be restored to class A when the plants die. Meanwhile, A is being aged or degraded to B as the year passes, and B is being degraded to C, so that 6 kg passes from form A to form B and 1 kg passes from B to C. Eventually all three are left as they were originally, as shown by the balance sheet of Table 2.2.

TABLE 2.2

Balance Sheet of the Three Classes

Class of supply	Delivered to plants, kg	Recovered from plants, kg	Reverted A to B, kg	Reverted B to C, kg
A	-10	+16	-6	-
B	- 5	-	+6	-1
C	- 1	-	-	+1

Plants have evolved over the ages with the ability to use very dilute sources of elements — to use solids of very low solubility. In this way the precious nutrients like P are conserved against removal by the rain and still may be sufficient for a good harvest. A well-known mechanism for cations is that of adsorption on the negatively charged colloids of soil, with only a small proportion being dissolved at any instant, the remainder being held, according to the scheme

$$\underset{\text{(solid)}}{M_nX} \rightleftarrows \underset{\text{(solid)}}{(M_{n-1}X)^-} + \underset{\text{(solution)}}{M^+}$$

In the above equation, M indicates a positively charged metal ion, and X represents a negatively charged colloid phase.

We may turn next to some of the heavy metals which have been recognized during this century as needed in small amounts for plants and animals, and which have had to be added to naturally deficient soils before the desired plants would grow; Zn and Mo have the closest analogy to P. Where Mo is needed for the growth of clover or other legume it is commonly applied much more generously than P relative to the plant's needs, so it may not be needed again for another 5 years, whereas P is needed annually during the stage of building up from original poverty. We may expect with Mo, as with P, to reach eventually — perhaps after 50 years — an adequate supply. With Zn there are many reports of the need for repeated applications, so that many kilograms per hectare are being accumulated. With Cu there seems to be little trouble in building up enough of what we might call a good second-class store. Mn represents the opposite extreme; on a deficient soil there is reason to believe that a good second-class store of 90 ppm Mn should be sufficient, but this is a huge amount to add and the more usual small amounts, up to 5 ppm (which represents 100 times the needs of a plant) have had very little residual effect. The residual effect of Co has also been very small.

Where an element threatens to accumulate in excessive amounts we welcome any inactivating mechanism. But such mechanisms are not welcome at the other end of the scale, which we are briefly considering here. If the added trace element rapidly becomes unavailable, one may do better than just to add it. First, one may change the soil. This alternative, which applies to Mn and Mo, has a bearing on our main interest in this book and should be considered here.

Manganese deficiency is a disease of neutral and alkaline soils, and provides a perfect example of "poverty in the midst of plenty"; a sensitive crop may fail altogether for lack of available Mn on a soil which contains 250 ppm, or 5,000 times the needs of the plant. Acidifying the soil to a pH of 6.5 or less will cure the deficiency. This may not be economically practicable, but it sometimes is, and sometimes where the disease has been caused by overliming one may restore a healthy situation within a few years simply by refraining from liming. Mo deficiency, on the contrary, is a disease of acid soils, and liming will commonly liberate enough Mo to cure it. There is no doubt that many of the great successes of the past in adding lime to soil have been due to this liberation of the trace element Mo.

A second alternative deserves only a mention here despite its practical importance; this is to add the missing element directly to plant or animal, while leaving the soil deficient. It is common to spray plants with a solution of the appropriate salt to overcome deficiencies of Fe, Mn, and Zn, and to treat Co deficiency in sheep by giving the sheep pellets containing Co. In the long run the sprays may add up to a substantial amount, but not in the short run.

Another alternative comes closer again to our main interest, namely to choose an appropriate species or variety of plant (Section 3.1). Many species and many cultivars have a particular ability to extract an element from an insoluble source, to exclude an element which may be toxic, or to tolerate an element which is present in unusually high concentration. For dealing with deficiency we look for the first ability; for dealing with excess we look to the second and third. This theme is considered at greater length later. The genetic differences among plants are so great that what is a dangerous accumulation of a foreign metal for one kind of plant may be harmless for another. We should expect to find, as we do, that soils are suitable or unsuitable for individual plants in terms of Zn or Cu or Ni just as they are known to be in terms of Al or Mn or Mo.

Moving our attention now to the extent to which soils inactivate elements which are already present in sufficient quantities for plants, we might begin again with P, the only major nutrient which is strongly held by soil and which therefore provides parallels to the heavy metals. In two soils to which heavy doses of P had been applied, one in the form of superphosphate for growing potatoes on a peaty clay, the other as liquid raw sewage used for irrigating a light clay, 1,100 kg and 4,300 kg/ha, respectively, had been accumulated in the top 10 cm over 50 years [1]. Another observation is that a soil kept under clover-ryegrass pasture for 20 years and repeatedly dressed with superphosphate had accumulated 150 ppm of easily extracted P in the top 2.5 cm and only 35 ppm in the next 7.5 cm, with the striking effect that when the topsoil was intimately mixed to a depth of 10 cm the yield of clover was lowered by 40%, the effect being entirely due to the loss of soluble P. We might say that a second-class supply had become third-class through this mixing [2].

All of this discussion should warn us against relying on figures for the total amount of an element in a soil. Sometimes we have nothing else to go on, and then we guess that the proportion of first-, second-, and third-class forms of any element is the same anywhere. If what we measure is in the fraction less than 2 μm, that is more relevant than the total and, in fact, that is what is often meant. Everything in that fraction is secondary — it has been in solution in that soil at one time or another. And yet while the smaller a particle is the higher the proportion of its atoms on the surface, it is easy to calculate that less than 1% of the atoms even in a particle of one-tenth that size (0.2 μm) are on its surface; and only the atoms on or very close to the surface can take part in a current season's activities. This warning is all the more important if one agrees that the root plays a positive role in extracting an element from some surface, and does not only wait for the appropriate molecule or ion to diffuse towards it.

2.2 GENERAL STATEMENTS ABOUT HEAVY METALS

While our 12 heavy metals will later be considered individually, some general statements may be made about them. First, all except Mo are primarily cationic in soils; Mo is anionic, occurring as MoO_4^{2-}, and must be considered separately. Cr may be added to a waste system as the chromate anion, but could not remain in such a highly oxidized state in a living system, so it will also be cationic* as Cr^{3+} (though this if in solution will be complexed, as set out below). Second, all cations of heavy metals have chemical features which on the whole favor their retention in soils. The chemistry of simple salts is traditionally taught in terms of NaCl and its closer relatives, the compounds of K, Ca, Mg in particular.

---

* The correct form of all these cations most of the time is as a hydrate, here $Cr(H_2O)_6^{3+}$. While the hydrated form is sometimes better used in print, especially for explaining certain reactions such as those referred to in this paragraph, it would be tedious to adopt it systematically in this book.

Yet about four-fifths of all the metals, including the heavy metals under discussion, form cations which have more complex chemistry [3]. They differ from Na^+ in being more "hydrolyzed" — reacting more with water to form hydroxy-complexes — and some of these complexes are dimerized and polymerized, as is well known for Al and Fe. Because of all this the heavy metals, as well as Al, are held more strongly by negative colloids than would otherwise be expected. At the same time, they form complexes with other anions, some of which are so stable as to move the metal into a negatively charged state. The most notable of such compounds are the chelates, organic compounds, some of which are extremely stable. These two properties are discussed below in their respective places.

2.3 THE REACTIONS OF HEAVY METALS WITH SLUDGE AND SOIL

The heavy metal from sewage treatment is divided between sludge and effluent (Section 4.1). The total amounts of metal applied to land are much greater with sludge; it involves a more acute problem so it will be tackled first. The small amounts in effluent have chemical reactions like those set out below.

The heavy metals added with the sludge may be in one of many forms of combination including oxide, sulfide, phosphate, or adsorbed by the sludge colloids.. After the sludge has been incorporated the new system — whether 10 or 50 parts of soil to 1 of sludge — will gradually reorganize itself. From time to time some of the metal ions will appear in solution; an oxide may be converted into soluble bicarbonate, or a sulfide may be converted microbially to sulfate. While many ions will long remain attached to colloidal particles of sludge, we may first consider the alternatives in front of any ion entering the solution. It may either (1) stay in solution and pass out eventually into drainage, (2) be taken up by a plant growing on the soil, which may later be harvested and removed, (3) disappear in the gaseous phase, or (4) be held by the soil in a temporarily or permanently insoluble form.

Disappearance in the gaseous phase (3) is possible for some foreign elements, especially arsenic and selenium, which form volatile organic compounds in some biological systems, The volatility of mercury and of some of its compounds introduces uncertainty into its balance sheets in soils. But beyond this mention we may ignore this possibility, which does not affect our central theme.

An example where both (2) and (4) are important is phosphate, which accumulates in the surface soil after application as fertilizer but may still be sufficiently available to supply all the needs of a crop. With the heavy metals it would be good if we could grow some inedible crop (say a fiber) which collected one or more metals and so allowed us to harvest them under (2), but the extent of such collection is generally trivial, and we aim at making the most of (4) and keeping both (1) and (2) to a minimum. This (4) will be our central topic in the following pages. As is discussed later, while the soil protects the plant under (2), both soil and plant take part in protecting the drainage under (1), so this path will not be pursued in detail.

2.3.1 Amorphous or Stoichiometric Forms

The emphasis in the succeeding pages will be on the removal of metals by adsorption, that is in a noncrystalline form. Other suggestions rely on precipitation as an exact or stoichiometric compound — carbonate or phosphate or silicate — involving a fundamental reorganization and recrystallization of some original adsorption complex, to give a simple formula like $BaSO_4$. Much of this discussion is inconclusive, and perhaps no exact solution to the problem is possible.

The attempt to fractionate the insoluble forms of each element into a number of exact compounds, each with its stoichiometric formula, is naive. It implies two questionable theories: one, that a formula like $FePO_4$ because it is exact gives a truer description than does "phosphate adsorbed onto hydrated ferric oxide"; the other, that calculations of thermodynamic equilibria are appropriately applied to the ever-changing colloidal and biological system of soil. Rather, since metastable systems are common in soils, an attempt at selective extraction of a soil for a particular compound may itself cause a shift of an element from one form to another, since the extraction telescopes a movement that would have happened during the next thousand years. So it was long ago observed [4] that the phosphate extracted from a soil with dilute HNO_3 decreases steadily with time of shaking, as the released phosphate alights on freshly activated surfaces of FeOOH and AlOOH. It might equally well be found that a heavy metal extracted with dilute HCl passes through a maximum and decreases as it finds new adsorption sites. The notion of exact stoichiometric compounds has a parallel in the common belief that the clay substances in soil are just like the pure crystalline minerals which are isolated from geological deposits or purified from soils. The alternative picture, which is favored here, makes more of amorphous compounds and surface effects. As an example we may note [5] that the adsorption of Co^{2+} on the colloidal soil mineral montmorillonite was doubled when silicic acid was added to the system — an effect that cannot be explained in the neat way that is used for montmorillonite, namely that it is a normal crystal which has a net negative charge because some Mg (with two positive charges) occupies places that might have been held by Al (with three positive charges).

2.3.2 Removal of Cations from Solution

Soil is almost a universal filtering medium which removes many of the elements which reach it in solution, substituting its own common ions. The first mechanism by which this happens is discussed here. However, two of our metals remain out of solution without using this mechanism, namely trivalent Fe and Cr, which are precipitated as hydrous oxides before reaching the land.

It is useful to give first attention to the removal of heavy metals by cation exchange. All soils contain negatively charged colloids. The inorganic colloid ranges from 0 (for a pure sand) to over 50% (for a heavy clay), with something near 20% being common for surface soils (loams, sandy loams, clay loams). Organic colloid varies in amount according to climate and management (see Section 4.6.1 for a detailed treatment of this), and commonly lies between 1 and 5% in surface soils, being less in subsoils. Both kinds of colloid carry a negative charge at the common level of pH (5 to 8); this charge is balanced by adsorbed cations, of which the common members in neutral soils are Ca, Mg, Na, and K, with H and Al being also prominent in acid soils.

Any added cations in the incoming solution enter into competition with those already in occupation, and if M^+ is the added ion and A^+ that originally present the reaction

$$\underset{\text{(solution)}}{M^+} + \underset{\text{(solid)}}{AX} \rightleftarrows \underset{\text{(solution)}}{A^+} + \underset{\text{(solid)}}{MX}$$

will go forward to an extent depending on the nature of M^+, A^+, and X^-, and the concentrations of M^+ and A^+, but some M^+ will stay behind at each site, so that it will be progressively filtered out as the water seeps through the soil.

The extent to which the negatively charged colloids can remove added cations from a soil is measured by its cation exchange capacity (c.e.c.); the whole soil is saturated with a convenient cation at pH 7 (commonly ammonium, though this may give misleading results, as shown below), all soluble salt is washed out and the saturating ion then leached out by another cation and determined in the leachate. The result is reported as milliequivalents (meq) per 100 g of oven-dry soil. (It is sometimes useful to multiply this figure by 10 and so to report "equivalents per million.") This figure gives the net effect of all the negatively charged surfaces, whether crystalline or amorphous. It varies among the different kinds of crystalline clay. For the common clay kaolinite it may be no more than 10 meq/100 g. Another common clay, illite, holds about 30 meq/100 g, and these two may occur together. For the organic matter of soil the value most quoted is 250 to 400 meq/100 g. For a whole soil, say a loam with 20% clay and 3% organic matter, one might estimate a likely c.e.c. of 11 to 12 meq/100 g, and such a value is common among surface soils. Much higher values (over 50) have been reported for soils with swelling clays; such soils would be powerful at holding the heavy metals, so might be sought after for our present purpose if their physical behavior were acceptable, but one does not count on finding such high values. These clays are stable only in the drier climates, while kaolinite (sometimes with illite) dominates in the wetter climates (where most of the world's large cities are).

A c.e.c. value of at least 15 might well be recommended as an insurance for a soil which is to be treated with sludge containing heavy metals, and this value will be used for the calculations that follow. As discussed later, one should expect the organic content to increase under sewage irrigation as well as under treatment with sludge, so that starting with the above modest value of 11 to 12 meq/100 g, one might well reach 15 at equilibrium. On this account the figure 15 was chosen for an ordinary soil in Table I (p. xv).

If we assume a bulk density of 1,330 kgm^{-3}, a hectare with a 15 cm depth of this soil weighs 2,000 tons so it has a c.e.c. of 0.30 ton-equivalent. The original places on this colloid are occupied by Ca, Mg, K, Na, together with Al and H if the soil is acidic. Assuming that all places were held by Ca^{2+}, this would mean 6.0 tons of Ca so held, the equivalent weight of Ca being 20 (half its atomic weight). It is instructive to compare this soil with a synthetic cation exchange resin. If such a resin had an equivalent weight of 150 (a very efficient figure) it would take 45 tons of such resin to do what this hectare does.

If now a heavy metal M is introduced, the reaction $M^{2+} + CaX \rightarrow MX + Ca^{2+}$ goes forward. The reaction is reversible, and if the pH is around 5.5, most of the bivalent ions of our heavy metals are not notably stronger competitors than Ca^{2+} for a place on the inorganic colloids. (The trivalent ions Fe^{3+} and Cr^{3+} are far more powerful, but as mentioned earlier they are so strongly hydrolyzed that they are omitted from this discussion.) There are individual complications to consider later, including oxidation for Fe^{2+}, Mn^{2+}, and perhaps Co^{2+}, and particular reactions with organic matter for Fe^{2+}, Co^{2+}, Ni^{2+}, and Cu^{2+}, so if we avoid these we have Zn^{2+} and Cd^{2+} to consider for the simplest case. The other bivalent ions share the simple part of their chemistry besides having their own peculiarities.

If we assume that Zn^{2+} equals Ca^{2+} in its competing power when pH is below 6, and that Ca^{2+} in solution is 1.5 mM (a common figure), then the equilibrium concentration of Zn^{2+} will be continually kept below 0.2 ppm (3μM, one five-hundredth of the Ca^{2+}) until the adsorbed Zn occupies 0.2 percent of the total negative spots occupied by Ca^{2+}, and so on in proportion. Thus most of the Zn^{2+} is immediately removed from solution, but it is not quite immobile, and both

Zn^{2+} and Cd^{2+} have been observed to move down below the plowed layer, while mostly accumulating in the surface. As explained in Section 2.3.3, this competition between Zn^{2+} and Ca^{2+} rapidly shifts in favor of Zn^{2+} as the pH moves from 6 to 7.

A few studies have been made using both Zn and other metals where the immediate retention of an added heavy metal has been measured, commonly using made-up columns rather than soil in its natural structure. (The natural soil would be too variable for this kind of study.) Where these have involved small amounts, as happened with the early work with deficiencies, these experiments have shown complete retention on the surface.

But this book is concerned with substantial amounts of heavy metals, not trace amounts. Retention has been measured on a substantial scale (together with evidence of downward movement with increasing saturation of the surface) at the metropolitan sewage farm [6] of Melbourne, Australia, where after 70 years of heavy irrigation on a light clay the Zn extractable with N/10 HCl at one site was: 0 to 2.5 cm, 438 ppm; 2.5 to 18 cm, 185 ppm; 25 to 45 cm, 43 ppm. Between 95 and 98% of these figures is additional Zn to that present in the unirrigated land, while the usefulness of this dilute acid as the extractant is shown by the fact that 80% of the total additional Zn in the soil was still extracted by the acid. (The total amount of Zn added over the years is not known, but the modest figure of 43 ppm in the subsoil suggests that it is far from saturation, so the little that has washed right through may here be ignored.)

Such a strong removal seems to call for a stronger mechanism than the simple exchange scheme just quoted, and for some of the metals the mechanisms are well known. Fe^{2+} is converted to the insoluble Fe_2O_3; and Mn^{2+}, while behaving like Zn^{2+} above in acid soils, is converted to the insoluble MnO_2 above pH 6; of the rest, Cu^{2+} and Ni^{2+} in particular are very strongly bound to organic matter. All these reactions and the peculiar reversion of Co^{2+} as well, are dealt with individually below. But the adsorption of Zn^{2+} itself is complicated by the fact that what is added to soils or to clays at pH 7 cannot all be recovered by leaching the soil with ammonium acetate, as Ca^{2+}, for example, may be. This kind of reversion calls for discussion here.

Our trouble is that the idea behind the word "exchangeable," which is simple for the four cations for which it was first developed (Ca, Mg, K, Na), is not simple for the heavy metals. Steenbjerg long since found [7] that adsorbed Mn^{2+} in a neutral soil could be displaced by Mg^{2+} in 20 times the amount that was achieved by Na^+, and NH_4^+ is closer to Na^+ than to Mg^{2+}, while Zn^{2+} is at least as difficult to displace as Mn^{2+}. Or one could quote Crooke's result [8] that added Ni could be recovered to the extent of 300 ppm with $ZnSO_4$, but only 17 ppm with K_2SO_4, K^+ being analogous to NH_4^+. Along similar lines is the work of Jones et al. [9] who chose $BaCl_2$ for extracting exchangeable Pb, which is especially resistant to the conventional replacing agents. Thus the figures reported for exchangeable heavy metals using NH_4^+ as the replacing ion may measure the first-class source, but by ignoring the second-class source extracted by more powerful cations they may exaggerate the degree of reversion, and may lead us to underestimate the potential uptake by plants. Besides the above examples we already know an element of which plants take up more than the "easily exchangeable" form of an ion, namely potassium, which is amply provided by some illitic clays from reserves untouched by NH_4 salts.

At this point we should query the quoted values for the c.e.c. of sludges and of soil-sludge mixtures. If they have been determined by the common method using an ammonium salt they will be too low because NH_4^+ cannot displace (at pH 7) the heavy metal that has occupied a place. One may be asked, Too low for what purpose? If the investigator wants to know how much NH_4^+ that sample can take up, he is using the right method. But if it is along the lines of our present enquiry, how far that sample's capacity to hold Zn is satisfied, the method is wrong. If the purpose is to measure the buffering capacity against changes of pH up or down, again it is wrong.

Thus, we cannot discuss adsorption of heavy metals onto soil colloids without discussing pH, which now follows.

2.3.3 Effect of pH

The most important single aspect of the reaction between heavy metals and soils is the effect of pH. Our heavy metals are held far more firmly — less reversibly — as the pH rises from 5 to 7. This fact takes us back to our earlier reference to the tendency of these doubly charged ions to hydrolyze to the form MOH^+.

Hydrolysis on a large scale, accompanied by precipitation, is characteristic for the trivalent ions Fe^{3+} and Cr^{3+} even more than for Al^{3+}. But the retention of the bivalent ions cannot be explained in terms of precipitating the hydroxide (which is too soluble). It is a question of adsorption, which applies generally to the negatively charged surfaces of the soil, organic and inorganic. The number of negative sites on the organic colloid increases strongly with pH, as discussed below, but this is not true of inorganic sites, and one should look for a general explanation.

Workers in other fields [10] have measured the adsorption of heavy metals (especially Co^{2+}) on colloidal silica (which also has a negative charge in suspension in water, and rivals the soil clays in its density of charge over the surface, 1 per 2,000 nm^2) and have found a great increase in adsorption between pH 6 and 7, just at the beginning of the range where the metal ion changes into the hydroxylated form ($Co^{2+} \rightarrow CoOH^+$). While the coulombic attraction of M^{2+} for the negative surface exceeds that of MOH^+, the effect is much surpassed by the contrary attraction of the doubly charged ion for water molecules keeping it in the water, and this is so even when the metal retains its primary sheath of $6H_2O$ or $5H_2O \cdot OH$. In this region where possible mechanisms are under lively discussion, a set of theoretical calculations for Co^{2+} predicts the rapid increase in adsorption found between pH 6 and 7, the exact value depending on the metal concentration. Ca^{2+}, on the other hand, shows no such effect until pH approaches 10 (Figure 2.1). One should then expect the competition between Ca^{2+} and Co^{2+} to depend on pH to a delicate degree around 7. The theory applies to any negatively charged insulating surface, but not where there is a specific reaction with the surface, as with organic colloids. The curves refer to solutions of 10^{-4} M, that is about 6 mg/liter for Co. For the more dilute systems with which we are concerned, the curves lie further to the left (lower pH) (Figure 2.2) and for any concentration a given proportion of Zn is adsorbed at a pH a little lower than for Co. Of the other two metals shown, clearly if any Cr^{3+} came into circulation it would be strongly held on soil colloids; but Cr^{3+} is more likely to be

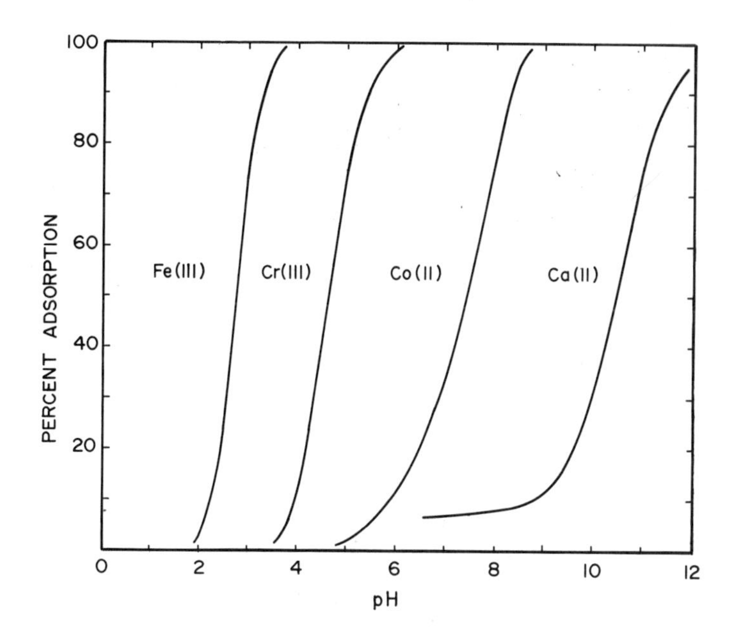

FIG. 2.1 Theoretical adsorption of Fe(III), Cr(III), Co(II), and Ca(II) on SiO_2 from 10^{-4} M solution as a function of pH. (After James and Healy [10].)

present, like Fe^{3+}, as the insoluble oxide, whether hydrated or not. At present one can only guess the extent to which Fe and Cr occupy sites normally available for exchangeable ions, and hope that no major mistake is being made by ignoring them.

This explanation is supported by the fact that N/10 HCl will liberate the heavy metal that has resisted the ordinary exchange reaction of leaching by a neutral salt. Insofar as the metal enters as the hydrolyzed ion MOH^+, a given number of sites can hold twice as many metal atoms as when it is doubly charged, so doubling the soil's protective power. This has long been recognized for Cu, which as $CuOH^+$ on the negative surface has an equivalent weight equal to its atomic weight. According to Vydra and Galba [11],

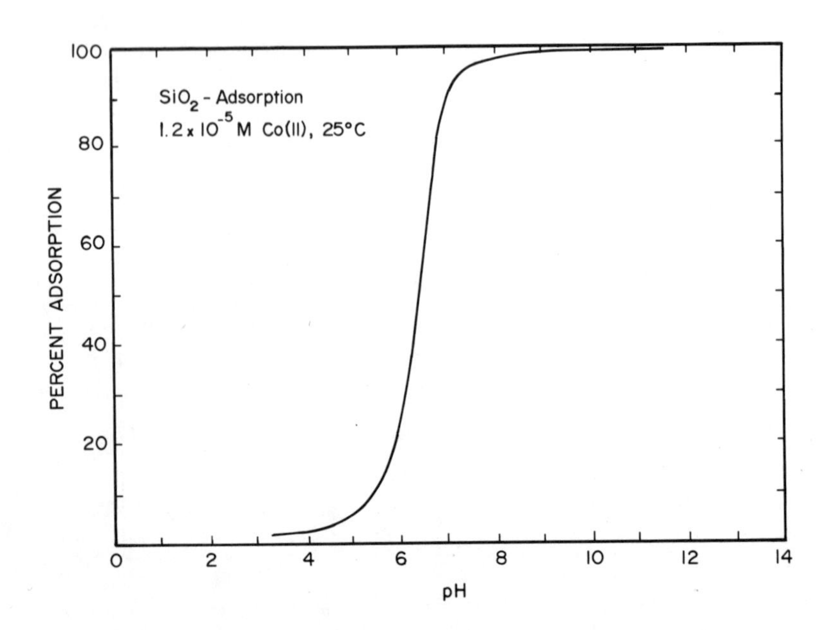

FIG. 2.2 Theoretical adsorption of Co(II) on SiO_2 from 1.2 x 10^{-5} M Co (0.7 mg/liter) as a function of pH. (After James and Healy [10].)

each adsorbed ion of Zn on silica releases one hydrogen ion, not two. But evidence for substantial adsorption of Zn as $ZnOH^+$ has not been found with soils.

This explanation has been strongly contested by some workers in the field [12]. For the present we can only record the general observation that not only Cu^{2+} but also Zn^{2+} and Ni^{2+} and Cd^{2+} become much less soluble and exchangeable by raising soil pH from 5 to 7.

The pH of a soil left to itself averaged over a year remains at the value which it has reached during its evolution. It oscillates during the seasons to an extent that is rarely recognized, depending on electrolyte content, leaching, incorporation of fresh organic matter, and microbial activity. However, some additions under the hand of man may incidentally change the pH. The best known example is ammonium sulfate, which through its conversion into HNO_3 plus H_2SO_4 has liberated Mn in toxic amounts in many parts of the world. The oxidation of organic matter may or may not change the pH, according to its total composition; thus nitrogen ends as nitric acid, so that pure protein free of metals is strongly acidifying, while carbohydrate ends only as CO_2 and when we include the common metals, a calcium organic salt ends as a base, $CaCO_3$ or $Ca(HCO_3)_2$. The mixtures present in sewage sludges, however, may include such anaerobic products as metallic sulfides, which will oxidize in soil to weakly acidic $ZnSO_4$ or to strongly acidic $Fe_2(SO_4)_3$. (Reduction is an alkalizing process while oxidation is acidifying, as is exemplified by the interconversions of NH_3 and HNO_3, H_2S and H_2SO_4, and the weakly acid Mn^{2+} oxidizing to MnO_2 and H^+.) Many sludges have been noted as having an acidifying effect on soils, an effect which might liberate abnormal amounts of Mn from the soil or of other heavy metals from the sludge. Such sludges might have been especially high in adsorbed ammonium.

2.3.4 Reaction with Organic Colloid

As quoted earlier, the organic colloid of soil has a far greater c.e.c., weight for weight, than the inorganic. It deserves special attention, therefore, as a retainer of the heavy metals. But besides its high c.e.c., it not only holds some heavy metals very strongly, but has specific reactions arising from its own chelating ability and the tendency of those metals to combine with the chelating groups.

The chemistry of the organic colloids of soil is still obscure. We assume here, as is commonly done, that while "raw" organic matter is highly variable, the more stable colloidal organic material, into which it has turned over the years in soil, has much in common through the world. This is sometimes called "humic material," a general term which makes no distinction among possible fractions (some refinement in the concept is discussed in Section 4.6.1). The source of the negative charge on the colloid is its carboxylate side-chains, together with many phenolic groups which can ionize within the common range of pH; since these phenols are weakly acidic the c.e.c. of the organic colloid increases substantially between pH 5 and 7. On a few sites some hydroxyls, and perhaps some imino-groups join with carboxylate in holding suitable metal ions in pentagonal or hexagonal chelate rings. The "suitable" metals are those of the well-known series, $Cu^{2+} > Ni^{2+} > Co^{2+} > Fe^{2+}$, with both Mn^{2+} and Zn^{2+} showing much less chelating tendency than their neighbors in the periodic table.

When the need of plants for Cu and Mn was first recognized, deficiencies were noted on peaty soils and it was believed that the organic matter was responsible for these deficiencies through its chelating power. This belief is questionable for both metals; for Cu, because Cu deficiency in organic soils is cured by adding Cu in amounts as low as one-thousandth of the c.e.c.; for Mn, because Mn^{2+} and Ca^{2+} compete on equal terms on the surface of organic colloid so long as pH is below 6 [13]. Yet it is true that Cu is very firmly held by the organic matter; the reason for the apparent anomaly, that the deficiency is easily cured, is probably that Cu can circulate in anionic form, as discussed below.

To sum up, the organic colloid retains Cu and Ni much more strongly than it retains Ca, and Mn, Zn, and Cd at least as strongly, though some would say "more strongly" of Mn, Zn, and Cd as well. An example of very strong interaction between organic colloid and Zn is the work of Himes and Barber [14], who saturated a reclaimed swampy sand with Zn and found that at pH 7, 2 meq/100 g was normally replaceable with K^+ and the remaining 10 meq only with Cu^{2+}, analogous to soils quoted on page 17; this firmly held Zn was also extractable with EDTA. They believe that all this firm holding was due to chelation with phenolic on top of carboxylic groups since the effect disappeared after treating the soil with methyl sulfate, which blocks phenolic groups. This is a very high estimate of the proportion of phenols in organic matter. If it were generally true it would mean not only that about 80% of the c.e.c. of the organic colloid is available for holding heavy metals, but presumably that the normal c.e.c. is thereby reduced by 80%. This article typifies the obscurity of the subject and the implications which are seldom brought into the open. A more general account of this subject is given by Gamble and Schnitzer [15].

2.3.5 Soluble Chelates

Most of our discussion of the chemistry of heavy metals in soils has centered on their removal from solution, and chelation was introduced earlier as a reaction with organic colloid removing a metallic cation. But the same kind of combination can have the opposite effect and so allow the same metal to stay dissolved. The word chelate denotes the gripping of a metal ion by two or more linked atoms to give a stable ring; it does not imply anything about solubility. Soluble chelates are formed between the heavy metals and small organic molecules, of which citric acid is typical and the most familiar. These soluble chelates generally carry a negative charge, so are not fixed on the generally negative surfaces of the soil. In fact, it seems likely that for any soil that is richly supplied with organic material and therefore with its biological products such as citric acid or amino-acid, the amount of any heavy metal in the drainage should be expected to reach a small minimum value, in the anionic or uncharged form. The existence of heavy metals in anionic form in soil has not been widely recognized until the last few years. According to one team working recently [16-18] not only is all the mobile Fe normally chelated and so either uncharged or anionic, but so is all the mobile Cu, most of the mobile Mn of neutral soils and up to one-third of the mobile Zn. This does not mean that we have been mistaken in emphasizing the fixation of the heavy metals as cations. This is correct; it is only a minute proportion of the total that is mobile, and it becomes mobile through its association with organic molecules which are themselves not very plentiful.

2.3.6 Effect of Phosphate

Additions of heavy metals to soils have usually been made in the presence of ample quantities of phosphate. Building up reserves of P is an early stage in improving agriculture, and applying the trace elements comes next in time. Zn deficiency in particular has occurred and continues to occur after adding ample P. Where sewage waste containing heavy metals is applied to the land, heavy amounts of P are commonly present. The question arises whether this phosphate may play a part in inactivating the excess Zn or other metals, as it has at the other end of the scale in inducing deficiency.

There is much evidence of antagonism between individual heavy metals and P, but the best evidence is that the antagonism is within the plant rather than within the soil. Some phosphates such as $Zn_3(PO_4)_2$ are too soluble to explain the disappearance of either Zn or P. At the same time, hitherto obscure minerals of very low solubility may yet be discovered in soils, such as the plumbogummites including crandallite $CaAl_3(PO_4)_2(OH)_5H_2O$ and gorceixite $BaAl_3(PO_4)_2(OH)_5H_2O$, one sample of which was found with 1% Cu [19]. One may conclude this topic by pointing out that one of the damaging effects of excess Zn on plants is a stunting due to P deficiency, and clearly this effect is avoided in highly phosphatic sludges.

2.3.7 The Ferric Oxide Theory

If the foreign heavy metals are to be specifically removed from circulation by inorganic reaction, it is presumably by adsorption on negative spots where the regular Ca and Mg do not go. One suggestion is that they are first adsorbed and later buried in the free ferric oxides of soil — this term including hydrated oxide such as goethite $FeO \cdot OH$, as well as the anhydrous form hematite Fe_2O_3. While the arguers for such adsorption [12] do not write the equation, it can only be: $2FeO \cdot OH + Zn^{2+} \rightarrow ZnFe_2O_4 + 2H^+$, where the hydrated ferric oxide has acidic powers which are not usually attributed to it — sufficient in fact to pull the Zn off the clay, though we have just seen that Zn adsorbed on clay can be very stable. This equation is consistent with the fact that raising the soil pH by one unit greatly strengthens the fixation of Zn (cf. Section 2.3.3). It is conceivable that compounds like this zinc ferrite would eventually crystallize and so bury the foreign metal; and we have the pedological evidence quoted in Section 2.6.1 that heavy metals are dissolved when free ferric oxide is selectively extracted. Yet what we have to explain is not the complete disappearance of the foreign metal but only its movement into a situation where N/10 HCl can still extract it — that is, into a difficultly exchangeable form — and one cannot see how the ferric oxide theory is specifically useful here. At the same time, at a pH approaching 7, ferric oxide develops an increasingly negative charge, so will add itself to the total negative surfaces.

A further theoretical drawback to this argument is that we are accustomed to think of goethite not as an acid but as a potential base which adsorbs phosphate and molybdate ions by exchanging hydroxyl. A more attractive side to this argument would be to keep the goethite as a base and let it react with anionic Cu (see Section 2.4.6), since Cu has been reported to be especially concentrated in free ferric oxides. The ferric oxide theory has recently become more popular and we return to it in Section 4.2.4.

2.3.8 Part Played by Subsoil

Most emphasis has been given here to the surface layers, where each seedling starts its life and where the most important reactions go on. However, the subsurface and subsoil can remove much of what remains in the solution as it descends after the reaction with the surface. If all of the uppermost meter plays its part before the incoming solution reaches the water table, these lower layers provide a much greater amount of clay colloid, though less organic colloid, than the surface. If the clay is kaolinitic — or if the soil is sandy — the c. e. c. may be no more than 10 meq/100 g, but even this taken over 1 m sums up to 1.3 ton-equivalent of the common cations which is potentially replaceable by the foreign heavy metal, so that if only 1% of the places are thus filled, 13 kg-equivalent is removed from solution. The filtering power of the subsoil will generally be greater than this. This line of thought leads to the principle that of the two possible kinds of danger through heavy metals — one that they will damage crops, the other that they will pollute drainage water — the crops are likely to suffer before the drainage.

This last point, however, might be considered without invoking the subsoil; if the crops are healthy, can the water draining away from their roots be seriously polluted? This question has not attracted much attention. However, plants and animals vary widely in their sensitivity, and some fishes are known to be especially sensitive to heavy metals, and this could be quoted in favor of some of the low limiting values that have been officially adopted.

2.4 THE MECHANISMS OF REMOVAL OF INDIVIDUAL HEAVY METALS

2.4.1 Iron, Chromium

These two metals are trivalent in soils. If Fe^{2+} is applied from outside, this valence is unstable at the ordinary pH range of soils and in the presence of oxygen; or if CrO_4^{2-} is applied, this higher valence is unstable in the presence of soil organic matter, so only Cr^{3+} need be considered here. With both these metals the hydrated oxide, often written $M(OH)_3$, has such a low solubility that this form is permanent in soils. $Fe(OH)_3$ may be reduced to Fe^{2+} only at very low pH by moderate reducing agents (a situation which does not concern us) or at ordinary pH by extreme reducing agents, which at pH 7 must be almost powerful enough to liberate hydrogen from water. Such reducing agents are produced in the treatment of sewage, when FeS is often formed. They are also produced in soils by anaerobic bacteria under prolonged waterlogging; excessive concentrations of soluble Fe^{2+} have been reported on flooding rice. However, this situation again does not concern us here. Fe is present in copious amounts in almost all soils other than pure sands; thus almost all soils, if they liberate soluble Fe^{2+} at all, will do so whether or not any Fe is added in solution, while in a normal aerated soil any added Fe, even if added as FeS, will soon be transformed into the stable hydrated oxide.

These two elements, Fe and Cr, are commonly mobile in soil only in minute amounts chelated with organic anions. The mechanism by which plants absorb Fe from soils is left obscure in textbooks; it involves local reduction to Fe^{2+} by the root itself. Cr has occasionally aroused interest as being possibly responsible for the poor growth of plants on serpentine soils, but this seems to be related to chromate in primary minerals, not to trivalent Cr. The toxic property of serpentine soil is usually explained in other terms, most often by excessive Ni. Since Cr is essential for human health, a moderate uptake by plants is desirable.

2.4.2 Manganese

Mn is one of the most plentiful components of soil. Therefore, as we saw with Fe, it is a priori unlikely that any application of the metal from outside would lead to excessive amounts in solution if the state of the soil did not anyway favor a liberation from the native supply. Two states of the soil can lead to excess soluble Mn, and we should consider these in turn.

The equation that connects the two major valences of Mn in soils (2 and 4) may be written conveniently in the two opposing forms:

$$2Mn^{2+} + 4OH^{-} + O_2 \rightarrow 2MnO_2 + 2H_2O \qquad (1)$$

$$MnO_2 + 4H^{+} + 2e \rightarrow Mn^{2+} + 2H_2O \qquad (2)$$

Equation (1) expresses the means whereby soluble Mn, whether native or foreign, is segregated as the insoluble MnO_2. This oxidation is carried out by soil microbes at pH of 6 or more, and goes well at quite low aeration, being favored by high concentrations of CO_2. Because this reaction is rapid, almost all Mn in soils of pH close to and above neutrality is insoluble. Equation (2) expresses the release of soluble Mn^{2+} from this store. The high ratio of hydrogen ions to electrons (2 to 1) shows that MnO_2 becomes a far stronger oxidizing agent — far more easily reduced — as the pH is lowered. Around pH 7, the organic compounds in the soil can react only slowly to produce Mn^{2+}, so the equilibrium amount through reactions (1) and (2) is very small. But at pH 5 the liberation through reducing agents (2) is far more rapid, while the microbial oxidation (1) is inhibited. Thus Mn^{2+} accumulates and enters into the same reactions as Zn^{2+} and related metals, as set out below. Its activity will be lowered by adsorption on colloids, inorganic or organic; but especially in sandy acid soils there may be enough in solution to damage sensitive plants, which include many of our staple crops. One major effect of liming acid soils is to lower the activity of Mn^{2+} by favoring action (1) and suppressing (2).

Acidity may liberate toxic Mn^{2+}, but so may a sufficient supply of electrons, even at a neutral pH. The commonest mechanism for such a liberation is by waterlogging, when the anaerobic bacteria produce strong reducing agents as noted under Fe. Plants that grow in waterlogged soil, such as rice, accumulate and tolerate in their tissues quantities of Mn as large as 1,000 ppm. We should add here [20] another possible way of liberating toxic Mn^{2+}, namely by sterilizing the soil, which inhibits the normal microbial oxidation (1) while still permitting steady reduction (2). This may happen not only by heating, as in commercial greenhouses, but also by drying in the sun, since bacteria are inactive when soil becomes drier than the wilting point, while the nonbiological reduction by the organic molecules of soil does not call for the presence of water. Any of these states of the soil — strong acidity or waterlogging or sterilizing — may produce sufficient Mn^{2+} to be toxic for most plants whether or not any foreign Mn is added. Normal management of soil avoids either state.

The damage which Mn^{2+} may cause, as with other heavy metals, is not well understood. One origin of damage is its antagonism to Fe; and it may sometimes likewise be lessened or removed by other antagonisms, as by heavy application of phosphate or by raising the intake of calcium, apart altogether from the common method of adding lime and so favoring reaction (1) above.

2.4.3 Cadmium, Copper, Nickel, Zinc

We introduced the preceding metals (Fe, Cr, Mn) only to dismiss their importance as additions to soil — one (Cr) because of its insolubility, the other two (Fe, Mn) because they are naturally present in high amounts and soils are already so managed, or cropping is so adapted, that they do not disturb us. But the above list of these four metals is different. They are present in normal soils only in small amounts, so that the addition of 100 ppm of one of the last three to soil (such as might come through adding 40 tons of sludge containing 5,000 ppm to a hectare-15 cm) creates a new situation. The examples where high concentrations of any of these are present consist either of abnormal sites where soils have been formed on metalliferous rocks, or of products of human action, where Cu or

Zn has been added to control pathogens or where waste products have been added to normal soil — this term mostly implying sewage wastes, though on rare occasions coal ash, a source of many rare elements, deserves a mention as a domestic addition to gardens. Serpentine has long attracted attention as a parent material giving rise to toxic soils, and Ni is the common offender here [8]. Other natural occurrences of toxic Ni have also been noted. Many observations have been made of peculiar growth or of unusual varieties of plants near ores of Cu and Zn, but most of the observations of both toxic Cu and Zn are related to human additions.

Cu and Zn have long been known to be essential for all living things; plants normally contain about 5 ppm of Cu and 40 ppm of Zn. We discuss here what mechanisms there may be in soils to keep the content at about those figures. Similarly, Ni and Cd, while as far as we know today they are not essential for plants, are harmless at their usual content of 1 ppm and 0.5 ppm, respectively, (see Table 2.3) and again we are concerned with mechanisms that hold them at such figures.

These four metals have some properties in common. They are foreign, they are bivalent, they are hydrolyzed, and they are potentially toxic. They will be separated here according to the ease with which they may be transformed into organic anions. Thus Zn and Cd, which are not easily transformed, may be first considered.

2.4.4 Zinc

Zn^{2+} has already been used in discussion as the typical foreign heavy metal, complex enough, but free from the additional complication of oxidation-reduction or ready chelation. For many purposes, it is usefully considered as analogous to Mg^{2+}. The two ions have a similar size, and Zn is well known to occur in ferromagnesian silicates in the positions normal for Mg. It is also taken up by many plants to the extent of many hundred ppm, as though there were no general mechanism at the root surface for distinguishing between it and the normal nutrient Mg. (One early explanation for the disappearance of Zn from circulation in a soil was that it occupied the position of Mg in a clay lattice.)

When small amounts (up to 10 ppm) of a Zn salt are added to a soil, one may follow its reversion over the following weeks. This was done, for example, by Follett and Lindsay [21], who added 5 ppm of Zn to soils of pH close to 7 and followed the diminution with time of the Zn extractable with the chelator DTPA: they found a decrease of 56% after 14 weeks in the greenhouse.

But when we consider adding large amounts (50 ppm or more) we have little reason to expect inactivation beyond being held in the adsorbing complex, with the additional tightness conferred by a pH of 7, if that is reached. This seems to be generally the situation. An addition of 650 ppm Zn is 20 eq/million, or 2 meq/100 g, and this might constitute 13% of places in a soil of c.e.c. 15 meq/100 g (Section 2.3.2) or 6% in a soil with 10% organic matter and no other colloid; these values for places occupied should be halved, to 6.5 and 3, respectively, if we accept $ZnOH^+$ as the form of the metal. In other words, the greater the amount of Zn added, the less reason we have to rely on queer unknown reactions to inactivate it.

2.4.5 Cadmium

While Zn is an analog of Mg, its relative Cd is an analog of the larger ion Ca. Roots take up Cd as though there were no separating mechanism from Ca. But the behavior of Zn and Cd in soil has much in common. While the amount of Cd in circulation is about one-hundredth that of Zn, it accompanies Zn in roughly proportional amounts through both adsorption and downward penetration. Where occasionally we have not the desired information about Cd we may estimate it from that of Zn. In one long-term study [22] most of the Cd applied to the soil over the years (in superphosphate) was exchangeable with neutral ammonium acetate. This evidence suggests that Cd was more mobile than Zn, seeing that its degree of saturation on the holding surfaces, whatever they were, was so low.

2.4.6 Copper

Cu is adsorbed on negative surfaces in soils like the other heavy metals. In two studies [23,24] that have been made of its adsorption on clay minerals and quartz, the adsorption from dilute solution has been shown to fit the Freundlich formula, $y = ac^{1/n}$, where y is the Cu adsorbed per unit adsorbent and c is the concentration of Cu in solution, a and n being constants. The adsorption is greatly increased on raising the pH, both in the above studies and in soils, so that the Cu is then more firmly fixed and thereby less toxic to plants. In this case there is little dispute that the ion $CuOH^+$ is the form adsorbed. We must note here that while added Cu is so strongly retained on acid soils that it barely moves towards the subsurface, it is still reactive enough to be toxic to plants.

In a thorough review [25], including the effect of applying bordeaux mixture to grape vines over 70 years, Delas cites a number of acidic soils which had accumulated about 500 ppm Cu of which from 50 to 150 ppm was exchangeable with ammonium acetate. This reagent can only underestimate the active Cu, showing that reversion here is not important. These soils had a c.e.c. close to 5 meq/100 g or 50 eq/million, so the saturation with Cu was between 1.5 and 4.5%. The fixation in the surface is generally so strong that the vines, with all their roots in the subsurface and subsoil, were unaffected, but when the vines were pulled out and annual crops sown these were badly affected. One profile is quoted which does not confirm the harmlessness of the subsurface, but emphasizes the degree of fixation, as follows: 0 to 25 cm, 200 ppm exchangeable Cu (using NH_4OAc); 25 to 50 cm, 74 ppm; below 50 cm, trace.

No figure for organic matter is quoted for these soils; it must have been low since the c.e.c. is low and the vines are kept cultivated.

Reuther and Smith [26] review damage by added Cu, again mostly as bordeaux mixture, in orchards in Florida where the trees were still growing. They too emphasize the importance of pH;

their soils were sandy, with a c.e.c. of about 5 mostly due to organic matter. At a pH of 6, they find that in general toxicity begins when total Cu reaches 5% of c.e.c.

Cu is strongly associated with organic matter. In normal soils it moves as a neutral molecule or an anion in organic combination, as it does inside plants. Such chelated Cu is much less toxic than is the cation; this point has recently been made in connection with marine algae, which are very sensitive to the inorganic cation but not to the normal marine form, which is the organic anion [27]. In another study [28] it was found that half the total Cu could be extracted from seawater with chloroform — that is, it was in uncharged organic combination. It is unfortunate that almost all our information about Cu in soils and cultures is derived from solutions of $CuSO_4$. At the same time, where Cu compounds have been added from outside, as in the French examples cited by Delas, there may well be cationic Cu in circulation, whether Cu^{2+} or $CuOH^+$ or some other inorganic complex; this is most likely in acid soils low in organic matter, such as these.

Colloidal organic matter is powerful at removing Cu^{2+} from solution, so where much organic matter is present we should expect that the only soluble Cu in equilibrium with it would be molecular or anionic, with the small organic molecule (perhaps a fragment of the colloid) competing with the large colloid for Cu. As stated earlier, organic colloid does not cause all Cu to be removed from solution so as to cause deficiency in plants. We know too little of the toxic properties and ease of absorption of anionic Cu to be able to assess how much the protection of plants by organic matter is due to retention of the element by colloid, how much to the absence of the cation. For an example of simple retention there is an experiment in which 1,920 ppm was added to a neutral peat in pots before oats and soybeans began to show damage [29].

There seems to be no evidence, as with Zn, that alkalinity reinforces the removal by organic matter. One should not expect it, since any strengthening of chelation by raising the pH will affect the soluble as well as the insoluble form.

The work of Kline and Rust [30], which seems to indicate that half of the Cu held in soil organic matter is mobile enough to be exchangeable with added labeled $CuSO_4$, is difficult to square with other lines of work. Their suggestion that mobile Cu may be estimated by extracting a soil with alkali, however, agrees well with the above discussion of anionic Cu.

2.4.7 Nickel

Ni behaves generally like Zn, though it forms stronger chelate links with organic groups and so has some analogies to Cu. But its main characteristic is to be held on the negative surfaces, the more strongly as pH rises. As with Zn, when an added Ni salt is equilibrated with a soil for a month, the Ni can be recovered only in small amounts with the conventional ammonium acetate, but this means little. More to the point is the observation [8] that soon after adding a Ni salt the NH_4OAc recovered 50% of the Ni, but if the soil was brought from pH 5.2 to 7.0 by adding lime, it recovered only 20%, which is in keeping with the lowered toxicity after heavy liming. The ability of organic matter to retain Ni up to 2,000 ppm has been tested using the growth of plants [29] (see Section 3.7).

2.4.8 Lead

The most surprising fact about Pb in soil is its apparent biophilic nature, namely its concentration in a profile in greatest amounts at the surface with the organic matter. This is the product of two causes: first, that some plants absorb it in substantial amounts; second, that it is very strongly fixed by soil. Aerial addition is heavy near highways, but could hardly be responsible for such concentration in remote forests. The fixation by soil follows the line already set out, namely that Pb^{2+} is hydrolyzed and polymerized, and is more inactivated as pH rises. In accordance with this tight holding by the soil, the Pb extracted with dilute acetic acid does not show the high surface values shown by the total figures [31], since this reagent is too gentle. But even Pb persists in a kind of exchangeable form, since 16% of the total Pb in agricultural (nonsludged) soils was found to be extractable with M/2 $BaCl_2$ [9].

2.4.9 Tin

It is interesting to consider how for generations we have plated iron vessels with tin, not only without disaster but without complaint. Tin has a rich chemistry, as is well known to every student of qualitative analysis, but this chemistry mostly lies outside the biological field. One may usefully compare it with two elements vertically related to it in the periodic table, Ti and Pb. On one side TiO_2 is so stable that one hardly thinks of it as having any chemistry. Tin also is very stable as the insoluble SnO_2, into which its bivalent salts are quickly converted. Lead differs from Sn and Ti in being stable in the valence of two, in which form it is toxic to animals. The similar low valence for Sn hardly enters the biological world.

2.4.10 Mercury

Such experimental evidence as we have of Hg shows that the metallic ion is strongly held by soil and is not absorbed by plants. The amounts of the element in circulation are far smaller than those of the major heavy metals considered here, so that mechanisms of adsorption within the soil will never approach saturation. It appears that most of the Hg in circulation in rivers is adsorbed on particulate matter [32] — that is, it is already out of solution.

2.4.11 Cobalt

Co^{2+} behaves generally like Ni^{2+} but is present in nature, as well as in industrial wastes, in much smaller amounts so that the mechanisms of adsorption in the soil never approach saturation. In keeping with this, where Co has been applied to soil in order to increase the amounts in pasture the uptake has been very small. In spite of this, plant collectors of Co^{2+} have been found, as discussed for example by Warren [33].

2.4.12 Molybdenum

Molybdenum has so far been excluded from discussion since it occurs only as an anion, which may be written here as MoO_4^{2-} although polymers also occur. Soils have no general mechanism for retaining anions; thus the anions nitrate, chloride, and bicarbonate pass through soil with no interference except for uptake by plants, while the cations which pass out with them are just those that are the most loosely held. However, there are particular mechanisms, namely when an anion forms a precipitate with an element in the soil or is adsorbed by a compound. The best known example is phosphate, which is removed from solution both on the alkaline side of neutrality by Ca, and on the acid side by Al and Fe. Molybdate is similarly precipitated on the acid side by Al or Fe, but not on the alkaline side, where it has often been reported as leading to "luxury consumption" by clovers and other stock foods, with an accumulation of as much as 90 ppm, which does no harm to the plant but is toxic to ruminants. If a soil is kept neutral to alkaline in order to inactivate any other heavy metals that may be added, any added Mo will be liberated from combination with Al and Fe; the possible interactions between it and the heavy-metal cations in the soil are unexplored country, but excess Mo in such a combination seems too unlikely for further pursuit here. While no such excess should be encouraged, Mo excess is often simply controlled by dosing the animal with copper, which the Mo antagonizes internally; Cu is likely to be in ample supply in plants grown with sludge.

2.5 ESTIMATES OF MOBILE HEAVY METALS

Thousands of papers have been written on the problem of estimating how much of any nutrient a soil will supply in the coming season.

Nearly all the studies relate to an element that is in short supply, usually potassium or phosphorus. Of the few studies relating to a possible excess, most concern manganese, but since excess Mn occurs (with few exceptions) on acid soils, the experience with it will not help us much. A fair estimate of toxic Mn can often be obtained by a simple extraction with water, whereas the problem before us requires a more sophisticated approach — to estimate not just what is soluble today, but what will become soluble during the next 3 months, or perhaps during the next 3 years. The most striking example of this approach, while not our problem here, is provided by nitrogen, which in organic combination may be completely insoluble yet may be destined to be liberated rapidly by microbial action.

Whether the question is of deficiency or excess, we should be clear that no exact answer can be given, since it depends on the crop and on the weather. If an exact answer were possible, perhaps we would not have had thousands of papers. The availability of any element in the soil depends strongly on temperature. The extracting solutions which are appropriate for the cool temperate regions of the world are relatively delicate, since the conditions suitable for releasing a bound element are short-lived; whereas more drastic extractions are needed to show the potentialities of the equatorial regions where the soil is warm and wet for 365 days and nights of the year [34]. Thus the danger of releasing a toxic metal increases as one approaches equatorial climates. But "availability" is also a function of the plant as much as of the soil, and this is more fully dealt with below. (This last statement may be found, among other places, in Mitchell's review [31].)

As a first step for estimating a cationic metal one may determine the amount in the exchangeable form — that is, immediately insoluble but capable of being easily brought into solution. Among the regular nutrients, potassium is commonly so analyzed, though like every element, it has its own complications. Among the heavy metals which may be in excess, this might be the first step. But we have already seen the difficulty of defining the term when used for heavy metals. On this account there is a good case for the common use of N/10 HCl as an extractant for the mobile heavy metals.

This is an especially powerful extractant, which will certainly dissolve the firmly held exchangeable metal but which may also dissolve some metal which has moved into forms beyond the exchangeable. In spite of this defect, the movement of both Zn and Cd downward through the soil has been followed using N/10 HCl [6] and N HCl [22]. One may feel assured that a supply of either of these which is not dissolved by N/10 HCl is no longer a possible threat either to growing plants or to a drainage system. But, like nearly all the traditional extractants for the major nutrients, this acid extracts many times more of the metal than the crop absorbs. (Suppose a crop of 10 tons/ha contained 100 ppm Zn, or 1 kg, and the acid extracted 200 ppm, or 400 kg/ha, then 1 part in 400 entered the crop.)

A further theoretical idea should be invoked for interpreting the analysis; namely, that the entry of the metal into soil solution or into a root depends not merely on the total amount in the exchangeable form but on its proportion among all the cations so held. This is a familiar theoretical principle, which has been invoked to explain Ca deficiency where the exchangeable Ca is apparently ample but where it is much outnumbered by Na and Mg (the other two major exchangeable cations of soils of pH above 7). In our case it might be suggested that Zn is harmless to all except a few sensitive plants so long as it occupies no more than 5 to 10% of the exchange sites; in other words, any Zn held in exchange positions is progressively more loosely held as the percentage rises above this range. However, this kind of interpretation must take account of the fact (Section 2.3.3) that the adsorption of the heavy metal rapidly increases between pH 6 and 7, while that of the competing ions (Ca^{2+}, Mg^{2+}) does not. Thus the critical figure for degree of saturation could well be 5% of c.e.c. at pH 6, 10% at pH 6.5, and 20% at pH 7.

This recipe is tentative. It combines two kinds of experimental information; one, that damage to sensitive crops has been reported when the Zn extracted by N/10 HCl has reached 5% of c.e.c.; the other, that a change of 1 unit of pH greatly affects this percentage figure. See, for example, Webber's work referred to later [35].

2.5.1 Other Reagents

After considering the meanings of "exchangeable" we may turn to two other reagents that have been widely used for comparing soils for their supplies of heavy metals. They illustrate the region in which thousands of papers have been published.

The first is half-normal acetic acid. This is not intended to measure the exchangeable cation, but rather the more reactive forms of the metal, whatever they may be. The acidity is weak (the final pH might be about 4.2); on the other hand, the acetate anion has some complexing tendency, so that the reagent extracts a fair amount of the mobile reserves of an element. One should realize that all soil extractions are arbitrary and inexact. Total figures, of course, are exact if the analyst is competent, but as already explained, total figures are usually not what we want. Rather, the value of an extraction (or a measurement like pH) rests in the correlation that it shows with other properties or behaviors of soil and plant. This constitutes the case for half-normal acetic acid; it has been used so much that one may interpret an extraction of a new soil much more usefully than one could with another reagent which was ostensibly more suitable but which did not allow one to compare with many other soils.

Finally there is the strong chelating agent, diethylenetriamine-pentacetic acid (DTPA) which (as a calcium salt) is much favored for estimating the heavy metal supplies available to plants rather than for identifying the form of the metal. By virtue of its chelating power it removes most or all of the exchangeable forms, depending on the metal and the system; and also dissolves many other compounds where the metal could not be called "exchangeable." Its supporters hope that not being acidic, it does not complicate the issue as does HCl by attacking fractions of the soil that are irrelevant for the enquiry; but this too is unexplored territory.

In order to illustrate the above theme that all soil extractions are arbitrary, we might here quote the reactive MnO_2 of soils [20]. This formula is used to include all the higher oxides of manganese in soils, which are insoluble, yet can react with reducing agents at pH 7. Thermodynamically all MnO_2 can be so reduced and dissolved. But at room temperature and with a mild reducing agent, soil A may deliver the whole of its 100 ppm Mn to solution in 5 minutes, while soil B delivers 1 ppm. With a stronger reducing agent, a lower pH, a higher temperature, and longer time soil B will deliver more and more until it eventually equals A at 100 ppm. The two supplies of MnO_2 differ in their state of subdivision and their crystallinity, A having smaller and more disordered particles. Plants take up ample Mn from soil A and may suffer from deficiency on soil B; but this difference can be brought out in the laboratory only by an arbitrary recipe which specifies the time and temperature and pH and the concentrations of reducing agent and electrolyte.

2.6 HEAVY METALS IN NATURE

Before discussing the reactions of the heavy metals of sewage with plants, one may recapitulate a few features of these metals in nature.

Trace elements in nature were noted from time to time during the nineteenth century, but could not be followed exactly since quantitative micro-analysis had not been developed; hence the name, elements that were recorded as present "in traces only." During the first quarter of the twentieth century, as analysis became refined, it was recognized that some trace elements were needed by plants or animals or both. The term has therefore some popular connotation of approval, which is unfortunate since a trace element may as well be harmful as beneficial — it is merely something that is conveniently recorded as parts per million, as is common for those trace elements, some desirable and some noxious, which we have assembled here as "heavy metals."

Many surveys have been carried out on the trace-element content both of economic crops and of plants growing wild. One compilation of such results is reproduced in Table 2.3, together with

TABLE 2.3

Typical Figures and Toxic Limits for Concentrations of Heavy Metals in Soils and Plants (parts per million, dry matter)*

	Soils		Plants	
Metal	Typical	Range	Common range	Toxic limits (using recent work)
Cadmium	0.06	0.01-0.7	0.2-0.8	100
Cobalt	8	1-40	0.05-0.5	—
Copper	20	2-100	4-15	30
Lead	10	2-200	0.1-10	—
Manganese	850	100-4,000	15-100	500
Nickel	40	10-1,000	1	25
Zinc	50	10-300	8-15	500

*First three columns of figures from W. H. Allaway, Adv. Agron., 20:235-271 (1968).

corresponding figures for soils. The last column in Table 2.3 presents some figures for contents at phytotoxic levels. These limits, like the normal contents, differ among plant species and situations.

Another such survey deserves a page of comment. Lounamaa [36] sampled great numbers of plants in Finland, ranging from lichens and ferns to deciduous trees and grasses, and separated leaves, twigs, and rhizomes and related their analyses for trace elements to those of the soils on which they grew. (The analyses are referred to the ash, not the dry matter of the plant; this makes comparison with other workers' results more difficult, but does not upset his main conclusions.) The soils were subdivided according to the rocky outcrop where they were sampled as either silicic, ultrabasic, or calcareous. While one should expect a wide range of values from such a survey (for example, the uptake of Mn and Mo varies greatly with pH, whatever the rock) the results are striking. The total content of many of the trace elements was higher in the plant ash than in the soil, often 5 to 10 times, and this occurred just as much for inessential elements (Ag, Cd, Pb) as for essential (Mn, Cu, Zn, Mo). The most notable case of the opposite was Cr, which was especially excluded by plants growing on soils from ultrabasic rocks. The result for cadmium — an element to be discussed at some length below — may be given both good and bad interpretation. Good, in that values of over 10 ppm in ash, so close to 1 ppm in the plant, were common; Lounamaa's figures like those in Table 2.3 show that natural levels of Cd are not as low as may be inferred from many other published figures. Bad, in that the element is very easily absorbed by plants, as recent experiments also show.

2.6.1 Prehistoric Pedology

It is worth while to consider what predictions about the future movements of the heavy metals may be made by exploring the evidence of the past, namely prehistoric pedology, meaning the study of soil in the field unaffected by human activity. This is the common meaning of the noun, which is here made explicit by my adjective.

An argument from prehistoric pedology might be invoked against the common practice of adding an element such as Mo to a soil on which plants fail for lack of it. It might be argued that such a practice is naive because the element is already present in the soil but has been converted over the ages to an unavailable form; so we must expect the added element also to revert to the same unavailable forms as were in the original soil. This argument is not convincing, partly because the reversion may take a long time and partly because the reverting mechanism may itself become saturated or upset by the fresh additions. We should now consider whether prehistoric pedology can help at all in the present problem of the reaction of soil with large applications of heavy metals. There are two lines of evidence, as follows:

1. The selective extraction of "free ferric oxide," a term that includes both hydrated and anhydrous forms of colloidal dimensions in which the iron is not bound as silicate either in clays or otherwise. (The term does not mean macroscopic grains of ironstone.) Such free ferric oxide may exist as a separate particle or as a coating. It is naturally very stable and any heavy metal incorporated within it would be very strongly held. Such free ferric oxide may be extracted only by very strongly reducing systems, one of which is oxalate under ultraviolet light [37], which breaks up the oxalate ion into short-lived fragments which reduce ferric to ferrous, while the excess oxalate holds the ferrous in solution as a complex. (Mitchell in reporting this work [31] omits the essential uv light.) This treatment, while it has little effect on clays, dissolves one-third of the organic matter, which must have shared with the Fe_2O_3 the responsibility for holding the reported amounts of 80% of the soil's Mn, 60% of the Fe and Co, 50% of the Cu and Pb, 20% of the Cr and Ni. But while the heavy metals may eventually be buried in the ferric oxides over the ages, movement towards them is likely to be very slow, and this does not seem to be a likely way of inactivating hundreds of kilograms per hectare of heavy metals over 10 or 20 years.

However, ferric oxides are more or less manganiferous, and any MnO_2 in the soil will be dissolved by this treatment (generally it is far more easily dissolved than Fe_2O_3). MnO_2 is especially well known as a scavenger of heavy metals, in particular of Co.

Pedological studies [38] have shown that most of the Co in a soil is bound with MnO_2 minerals; and in this case the short-lived experience of 1 year [39,40] agrees with the pedological finding, since Co applied as fertilizer to a manganiferous soil on deeply weathered basalt in Tasmania became unavailable to pasture plants and so failed to cure the Co deficiency of sheep which is endemic to this area. There are good grounds [41] for believing that what favors this binding is the oxidation of Co from valence 2 to 3.

Perhaps we should link with these studies the comparisons made by Mitchell [31] between well-drained and poorly drained sites, where the poorly drained showed much higher values for heavy metals extractable with N/2 acetic acid. If the drainage became good and ferrous and manganous ions were oxidized, these heavy metals would be trapped in the resultant oxides.

2. The distribution of elements down a profile [42]: This is the product of many processes, of which we mention here clay formation and destruction, leaching, and uptake of plants and deposition as litter at the surface. If an element is present in greater amounts in the surface horizons than in the subsurface or subsoil, this indicates that it is both used by plants and held by soil against leaching. Among the major nutrients P shows this double effect, and still more so if one measures total P per unit of clay, when the surface may show 10 times the concentration of the subsoil. Among the heavy metals (here excluding Fe but including Mn) there may be more total metal in surface than subsoil, and examples may be found for Mn and Zn, but for many profiles there is surprisingly little difference for most metals, so that we get little help here, beyond the common concentration of Pb in surface horizons, as noted in Section 2.4.8. However, this line of work is thwarted by the fact that many of these profiles are young enough to contain large reserves of trace elements in the primary minerals, and these are uniformly distributed.

On this second score we meet an earlier warning against putting too much faith in thermodynamics — a theme argued at length elsewhere by Morgan [43]. In other words, is our time-scale in terms of years or of thousands of years?

CHAPTER 3

RELATIONS OF PLANTS TO THE HEAVY METALS

We have up till this point considered chemical aspects of some heavy metals added to soils, in particular their removal from solution. Clearly if they were not removed almost entirely from solution the land could not be cropped. But an element may be present on the solid phase of the soil and still be taken up by some plants in abnormally high amounts, and this will be considered next. Only five of the 12 heavy metals originally introduced, namely Zn, Cu, Ni, Pb, Cd, are further followed here. As explained earlier, Fe and Mn are common in soils, so their introduction does not set a problem. Cr enters into soil solution in only minute amounts; while Co, Hg, Sn, and Mo are very minor constituents of sewage wastes, and the first three of these are thoroughly inactivated by soil.

Before turning to the full complexity of the system of crops grown on sewage sludge or effluent in the field, it is useful to review some simpler systems. First one must realize that plants differ greatly among themselves, and this point must be always in front of us. But with any plant we may begin with a simple system where the heavy metal is added experimentally to a solution or to a soil. The culture solution, as is explained below, is a long way from our full complex problem. Plant cultures, whether in pots or in plots, where a metallic salt is added to a soil, may give valuable information, but this treatment is far more damaging than the addition of the same amount of the metal in sludge, both because the soil is not being protected by accompanying organic matter and phosphate and because time is required (and may not be given) for the added metal to reach a less active though still metastable state in the soil. But these simpler experiments will help in interpreting the field experiments and experiences which are the center of this second part of the book.

3.1 DIFFERENCES AMONG PLANTS

One major theme in this book is the opposite to the common introduction to plant physiology. One begins by learning the properties that are shared by all plants, namely the processes and cycles of the major nutrients and the functions of the trace elements (Mo for nitrate-reductase, for example). But for our present purposes we shall stress the differences among plants, both in their tolerance for foreign elements and in their ability to exclude them. Plants differ here, not only between genera and between species, but between varieties of the same species, where a single gene may be responsible for the difference. We may introduce the topic with two universally present elements, silicon and aluminum.

Of the two major groups of higher plants, the monocotyledons, which include the grasses and the common cereals, absorb silicic acid in the transpiration stream, so that one may calculate the water transpired by analyzing for the silica in the plant and the silicic acid in the soil solution [44]. The other group, the dicotyledons, generally contain less than half as much silica; they have a mechanism for excluding it. Coming to aluminum, plants differ greatly in their content. While it is often below 0.01%, the hydrangea has been recorded as having 1%; when growing on acid soils with a high intake of Al it produces blue flowers (the blue being a compound of its normal pigment with Al), while on neutral soils the flowers are pink, the normal pigment. Many high-Al plants belong to wet climates, especially to tropical climates, and values as high as 7% in plant tissue are recorded [45].

The introduction to the heavy metals on this theme is the field of biogeochemistry, where one can be led to metallic ores not only by analyzing plants to determine whether an unusual element is present in high amounts, but also by looking for particular species which are known to concentrate an element.

Some extreme examples of tolerance have been recorded. There are the special plants of mining areas [46,47], such as colonial bentgrass (Agrostis tenuis) existing near Pb, Cu, and Zn mines; the calamine violet, (Viola calaminaria), of Zn mines, and the healthy larch and black spruce described by Dykeman and de Sousa [48], as living in a swamp of cupriferous peat (over 1% Cu), and containing about 500 ppm Cu. Warren in reviewing his achievements in searching for ores by analyzing plants [33] quotes a hemlock (Tsuga sp.) with 3.4% Cu in the ash of its leaves, which might mean 1,700 ppm or more in the dry matter.

There are many plants that accumulate an element which is normally considered toxic to living things, yet do not themselves suffer. Two well-known examples of such accumulation are those of Se by Astragalus spp., reaching 1.5% in dry weight, and of Mo by clovers, reaching 90 ppm. The first figure is lethal for grazing livestock, the second causes serious illness in dairy cows. Both of these examples occurred on calcareous soils that were unusually rich in the respective element. A less known concentration of a toxic element is the figure of 0.5% Ba for the brazil nut [49], apparently a concentration from no more than normal sources in the soil. It is curious that soils contain large amount of Ba, a fact which has never disturbed us; most of the plants that concentrate it (which include some trees) are not used for food. The brazil nut either has a mechanism of competing against the soil, or has not developed a mechanism for excluding Ba from its flower.

At the other end of the scale, where soils have been cropped and have shown acute deficiencies of Fe or Mn, for example, with the imported crop, there has always been a characteristic native vegetation which thrived on those soils. In recent years there have been studies of varietal differences, for example of a soybean [50] which can obtain its necessary supply of Fe from a soil on which another variety succumbs to chlorosis. So a policy of breeding the appropriate plant, rather than changing the soil, has recently appeared [51], in order to deal with either deficiency or excess in nature.

The biogeochemist looks for the plant that tolerates a particular metal. Such a plant may have a high concentration, such as those quoted; yet in the mineralized country described by Nicolls et al. [52] at Cloncurry, Australia, each successive species prevails in turn in terms of its ability to exclude, even though it may be an accumulator at the upper end of its range.

Here are two properties in which plants differ, namely (1) the amount of metal absorbed from a given source in the soil, (2) the concentration in the tops at which the plant is damaged. (The damage may begin in the roots, but we rarely have this information.) To these a third must be added, (3) the movement of the metal into flower and seed. Of the metals discussed in this chapter, (2) is foremost for Zn, Ni, and Cu, while for Cd we are more concerned with (1) as possibly leading to toxicity to animals, though a low value for (3) may also decide on the choice of a species or variety in practice. Generally the heavy metals under discussion are concentrated into leaf or straw, in amounts that vary greatly with the part of the plant and its age, while the amount of the metal in the seed is more stable and less dependent on the soil.

3.2 ANTAGONISM

We are poorly informed about the nature of the damage done by excess heavy metals and therefore about the mechanism of resistance. One kind of damage consists of antagonism. The full mechanism of antagonism in plant physiology is beyond our present scope, but we may consider two kinds. First, that of heavy metals to phosphate, which may be thought of as mutual precipitation within the roots. This is certainly one source of damage by both Zn and Mn, but this at least should be avoided by the highly phosphatic sludges. Second, the antagonism of heavy metals to one another, which may be thought of as competition for a place on some compound such as an enzyme. Patterns of iron or manganese deficiency have been observed on plants given heavy doses of Zn, Ni, or Cu. Some of the damage done by excess Mn is cured by a spray of $FeSO_4$, as is commonly done for pineapples, for example at Hawaii. In an experiment in poor gravelly soil in Western Australia the following successive strips of oat plots were seen: (1) with superphosphate alone, the dark colors of Zn deficiency; (2) with super and zinc, the wither-tip of Cu deficiency; (3) with super and zinc and copper, the gray-speck of Mn deficiency. An example of such antagonism in practice is quoted later (Section 4.2.2).

The theme of antagonism should be kept in mind in reading the different figures quoted by different authorities for toxic limits for the several metals. These limits depend partly on ratios to other elements. For example, Mn in a healthy plant should be at least 15 ppm (some might quote 20 ppm). Many plants tolerate 10 times as much, but damage from excess is common at 300 ppm. Where apples and pears are damaged by Mn, the ratio Mn/Ca appears to be important; the more Ca in the tree, the more Mn can be tolerated. Perhaps something similar happens with Ni, which often occurs in plants at 2 to 5 ppm. Plants damaged by excess Ni — those growing on serpentine soils, for example — have been recorded with 50 to 80 ppm Ni. Yet after heavy liming, the plants on these soils grow normally again, but still contain heavy amounts of Ni (50 ppm) [8].

This warning about antagonism applies equally to animals. For example, the high Cu content of sludge might be an asset in animal feed if it led to increased Cu in plants by virtue of antagonizing at least two other metals, namely Cd and Mo.

3.3 INFORMATION FROM SIMPLIFIED SYSTEMS

3.3.1 Culture Solutions

Experiments in culture solution have been aimed at marking the limiting concentration at which a heavy metal decreases the yield of a plant. They may either over- or underestimate the damage to be expected from a given concentration.

1. Underestimate, as appears from work with flowing culture. In conventional culture work the root exhausts the solution in its vicinity as contrasted with a soil, which may keep the concentration steady. Flowing cultures, on the other hand, constantly replenish the solution, and lead to surprising conclusions that adequate or dangerous concentrations occur at one-tenth of the values found in conventional cultures, for example, with micromolar Zn [53].

2. Overestimate in at least three ways:

   (a) The heavy metal has always been added as the simple salt. But in the soil the heavy metal is partly present in chelated form, and so is less toxic. In the absence of extensive experiments where chelated elements are added to plants one can quote again the two oceanic reports cited in Section 2.4.6.

   (b) The soil solution contains silicic acid, commonly between 10 and 30 mg/liter. Vlamis and Williams have shown [54] that this greatly ameliorates the toxic effect of soluble Mn on barley, by a mechanism as yet unknown. This may well be true also for other heavy metals and the generally greater tolerance of heavy metals by the Gramineae may be related to their high Si content. Perhaps Bowen's work [55] with sudan grass supports this idea for Zn and Cu, though he added his Si as Na_4SiO_4 solution, not as $Si(OH)_4$, and one cannot be sure how much Cu or Zn was thus precipitated from solution, especially since he used strong solutions of 3 or more mg/liter.

   (c) The uptake of any element is affected by competition or antagonism and the culture can hardly reproduce the situation in the soil. There are many rival formulas for cultures, and one should expect them to give different results for threshold toxicity for any metal. Ammonium is incorporated into some recipes in order to keep the pH low enough to avoid precipitating Ca phosphate, not in order to simulate the field. In comparing the two forms of nitrogen at the same steady pH, giving nitrogen all as nitrate ensures that bivalent cations are more easily absorbed, while giving ammonium may suppress them.

The question whether heavy metals should be supplied in inorganic or in chelated form has hardly been discussed. Iron is commonly supplied as chelate, as a convenient way of ensuring that it stays in solution at least a few days; the others are commonly supplied as simple salts. Yet there are difficulties in both directions. If any metal is supplied as chelate, it may not hold a monopoly of the ligand that was used; so the effect of adding Fe as citrate is that some Cu and Zn, for example, will also be present as citrate. At the same time, as already pointed out, a metal which we know is normally chelated in soil is not fairly represented in culture as its simple ion. A further difficulty arises when the metal is added as a synthetic chelate like EDTA or DTPA, namely the possibility that this may enter the plant and alter the transport of one or other metal inside the plant.

With all their drawbacks, experiments with solution culture (or with sand culture) are necessary to give background information. For example, we know from such experiments [56] that many plants will readily take up Cd from 0.01 mg/liter solution into their tops, which they do not do with Pb; further, that the uptake of Cd is much diminished if normal amounts of Ca and Mn are simultaneously in solution.

3.3.2 Pot Tests with Soil

At the next stage of complexity, where plants are grown in pots of soil, the concentration in solution of the element under study is not known and is not under the experimenter's control. The soil is uniformly mixed in order to reduce variability. This has to be done, but the process destroys the natural structure, and the packing of pots is a perpetual problem. This alone marks a serious departure from the field. But not only do the water regime and the root system differ from those in the field, but so commonly does the temperature, sometimes strongly. Now we cannot do without pot tests. Many of the experiments quoted in the following pages were carried out with pot tests, and some of them (for example, studying the effect of mixing the soil with 100 ppm cadmium as CdO) could not have been carried out in the field. Yet one must be cautious in extrapolating results from pot to field, for the reasons here given as well as those given at the introduction to this chapter. In one experiment already quoted [22] the Cd content of subterranean clover grown in pots was two to three times that in the field. There is good reason to suspect that such an exaggerated effect is common for the heavy metals.

3.4 UPTAKE AND TOLERANCE OF ZINC

Zinc comes first in all our discussion, as the metal that stands for the rest in its chemistry, as the one that occurs in the highest amounts in sludges, both domestic and industrial, and as one that is the most difficult to put out of sight and out of mind. It may be thought of as intermediate between the major nutrients and the micronutrients. If fact, there is no clear line between these two groups. The distinction commonly made between them is partly a historical accident, in that we could not recognize that zinc was essential so long as analytical work was confused by its presence in glassware in laboratory work and as an alloy in blocks in distilling water. But zinc is of major importance in many fields of agriculture and is applied as fertilizer more widely than is magnesium. We should find it easy, therefore, to think of it as beneficial; it is likely that mankind would be healthier if we had more of it in our food.

There are few reports of damage to plants by excessive Zn in soils. In some of these, inorganic Zn was added and the soil given no time to equilibrate as would happen in the field under rain and irrigation. Perhaps Webber's report [35] best sums the situation. In this experiment, carried out in the field, 20 eq/million of zinc was added as $ZnSO_4$ to a "brick earth" and wheat was grown with and without liming. At pH 6.5 no damage was done; at pH 5.5 the yield was reduced to 20%. Thus on the acid soil the colloids hold the metal too loosely to protect the plant, but near neutrality the mechanism is efficient. We are not told the c.e.c. of the soil but it was probably at most 20 meq/100 g (or 200 eq/million), so that at pH 6.5 the soil successfully held Zn amounting to 10% of its c.e.c., and this is probably the best way to use such a result. Another suggested boundary for toxicity is given in the same article as being endorsed by the British Agricultural Development and Advisory Service, namely 125 ppm of Zn soluble in N/2 acetic acid, a figure that is difficult to relate to the first one; one would guess that more than 125 ppm of the additional 640 ppm would have been dissolved by the acetic acid.

It would be most important to know whether there is any limiting value of pH beyond which Zn can do no harm. Certainly plants continue to absorb Zn in high amounts at pH over 7 (for example, the collector Swiss chard appears with 630 ppm); but there is little evidence of damage beyond an experiment in a phytotron [57] on a soil of pH 7.5 which was treated with $Zn(NO_3)_2$ and not leached. Many species of plants were stunted by this treatment (indicating a deprivation of phosphate), but it is difficult to apply the experiment to the field. However, again plants took Zn from this alkaline soil up to 300 ppm of their dry matter without being damaged.

High amounts of available Zn in soils may lead to high figures for Zn in plants, much more in the vegetative parts than in the seeds. In an experiment representative of the 1970s, Boawn [58] reports several leafy vegetable crops, grown in the field, accumulating 300 or even 400 ppm without damage when Zn was added up to 0.9 meq/100 g of a soil of pH 6.1. Of the 12 crops grown, only Swiss chard and spinach were damaged at this high rate, and Swiss chard in particular was a collector, ranging to over 800 ppm Zn. One should be prepared to find a range of Zn concentration as great as 5:1 in comparing two plants growing on the same soil. Experiments such as this have shown that some earlier figures quoted for the upper tolerable level for Zn content were far too low.

It is unlikely that animals have been damaged by eating plants that have accumulated much Zn, as here. According to Underwood [59], 1,000 ppm Zn in diet may be harmful, but even at this level the experiments were done with inorganic Zn, and perhaps plant Zn behaves differently in the digestive system.

3.5 UPTAKE AND TOLERANCE OF COPPER

As stated earlier (Section 2.4.6), Cu is damaging on soils of low organic content to a degree depending on the pH. On acid soils an exchangeable Cu (with NH_4OAc) 3 mol% of c.e.c. was damaging while on neutral soils damage was slight. Delas [25] quotes a case on a soil containing 80 ppm exchangeable Cu where spinach was cured of Cu toxicity on bringing the pH from 4.7 to 5.9. In a recent paper [60], damage at about 3 mol% of c.e.c was reported with snapbeans (Phaseolus vulgaris) on a loamy sand of pH 6.7 treated with $Cu(OH)_2$. This seems to be the lowest acidity on record for Cu toxicity.

On soils of high organic content, besides the already quoted cases of tolerance in nature, there is an experiment with neutral peat [29] where additions of Cu below 1 mol% of c.e.c. (1,920 ppm) were harmless, but at this level or above were damaging to soybean and oats.

The Cu content of normal plants, even with high applications of Cu, rarely exceeds 30 ppm unless damage has been done (some workers would say 20 ppm). Thus it accumulates less easily in plants growing on metalliferous soils than do Zn and Ni. The Cu in seeds does not increase with addition to the soil.

3.6 UPTAKE AND TOLERANCE OF CADMIUM

Cadmium has aroused concern less as a possible reducer of yields than as a possible contaminant in food, and on this account it warrants a longer discussion here.

For trace elements in general, some workers start with the assumption that all living things are equivalent; if the plant can tolerate so much of the metal, so can an animal, or if a bacterium can tolerate it so can a higher plant. A convenient example of the principle is zinc, which will damage or kill a plant before it accumulates in amounts dangerous to an animal that eats the plant. The idea may have two bases; one is biochemical, that living things share the same mechanisms, the other is evolutionary, that exposure to the metal over the ages has compelled organisms to deal with it or die. Thus one might feel reassured by the fact that the city wastes are decomposed by bacteria in spite of the heavy metals; if bacteria can segregate or exclude them, so should the higher plants. Yet the reassurance is not justified, at least with Cu and Cd, since these elements may initially inhibit the first generations of bacteria so that digestion is temporarily held up, but we cannot achieve such a rapid selection among the higher plants, which will require many years as contrasted with the bacterium's few days. (Partly for this reason, partly for economy in space, the interactions of microorganisms with heavy metals are not further discussed in this book.)

While zinc provides the happiest example of the above assumption that all living things are alike, cadmium provides one of the unhappiest examples of the opposite, in its ability to accumulate in a healthy plant in a concentration dangerous to the animal or human consumer. The evolutionary argument of the preceding paragraph has been expressed in the form that the toxicity of an element is inversely related to its abundance in nature. One can find elements which illustrate this idea, such as beryllium or mercury, though it must not be accepted literally - thus the toxic barium is plentiful in nature. The idea has been especially invoked for cadmium, which is naturally present through the world in only minute amounts so that its recent invasion via industrial wastes poses new problems for living things. The work of Lounamaa [46], on plants growing wild, quoted on page 41, throws some doubt on how new the problems are; but apart from this the above idea, while attractive, is not quite sound. The animal body has learned to protect itself against cadmium by producing the specific molecule metallothionein. It seems that cadmium has always accompanied zinc through natural systems in a proportion of one to one or two hundred.

3.6.1. Limits to Safety in Food

Regarding animals in general, Underwood [59] quotes 100 ppm Cd as a tolerable concentration in food. As he points out, the tolerance for any toxic element is much increased if antagonistic elements are also present in the food, and zinc, calcium, and selenium are all effective against cadmium. On the other hand, recent work with sheep [61] has shown that levels of only 12 ppm Cd in food will upset the copper metabolism; how far this may be remedied by giving additional Cu is not stated.

However , experiments with animals are short compared with a human lifetime. Cadmium accumulates in the body, so that a given intake which may be harmless over 1 year may be dangerous over 20 years. Thus a new problem arises over permissible levels in human food, and here opinions differ.

The most alarming evidence that is quoted about chronic cadmium poisoning is its appearance as the "itai itai" disease on the Jintsu River in Japan [62], where about 100 people have been crippled and have died prematurely. The sufferers are all of middle age or older, and the disease has been traced to the 1940s, when the river was contaminated with waste from a mine upstream and the mud of the rice fields was also contaminated with metals. Whether the present daily intake of the inhabitants, namely 600 μg cadmium, will lead in later life to the disease is only conjecture, but the average daily intake in Western countries is only 60 μg.

Most human diets contain about 1 part of Cd to 100 of Zn, which is essential for animal and plant life. While no exact calculation is possible here, this line of thought suggests that mankind's necessary intake of Zn has always involved an intake of Cd of at least the quoted figure of 60 μg daily. Obviously our bodies can take care of this. It is sensible to choose one's diet so as to be sparing of foods that concentrate Cd, notably kidney and liver and shellfish. (The situation is somewhat similar to that of Hg in the large pelagic fishes, shark and tuna and swordfish, which naturally concentrate Hg through the food chain to levels which might be dangerous to humans if they ate nothing but these fishes.) But it would be unreasonable to require that no food should exceed the average concentration of Cd, namely about 0.05 ppm. Perhaps an upper limit of 0.5 ppm in a major item in human food will turn out to be safe, especially when one considers all the antagonistic elements (Ca, Se, Zn) and the fact that no other element is known for which such great differences are recommended for intake by mankind and domestic animals. Some minor items (such as kidneys) will remain with much higher levels of Cd than this [62].

3.6.2 Uptake of Cadmium from Culture Solution and in Pot Tests

It is clear that roots take up cadmium rapidly from culture solution and that some plants accumulate large amounts in their tops. Thus with a flowing culture of 12.5 liters containing 0.01 mg/liter Cd, miscellaneous plants had absorbed all the cadmium within 3 days, and perennial ryegrass had absorbed half of the cadmium from 0.25 mg/liter Cd, also in 3 days. The uptake is much reduced by the competitive ions Zn, Mn, and Ca when present in 40-fold excess such as would be expected in any soil. When the movement from roots to tops was followed it was found that most species of plants when given a normal supply of phosphate retain at least 70% of the cadmium in their roots, though this ratio varies among species. Amounts of the order of 40 ppm of dry weight were found in the tops of many plants in this culture work, without any visible damage [56].

The work of Page, Bingham, and Nelson [63] was aimed at determining the concentrations at which plants were damaged, which is not our main concern here. Some of their figures are very high; using 0.1 mg/liter Cd added to standard (not flowing) culture solution they found 280 ppm in the tops of red beet (which was sensitive to damage) while sweet corn (which was tolerant) gave 90 ppm in the leaves. A more striking demonstration of accumulation was unintentional. The control solution contained 0.0005 mg/liter Cd from some of the reagents used, and even from this the crops collected a few micrograms, the cabbage having 0.75 ppm in its leaves. This work may have been affected by the fact that excess of the chelating substance EDTA was present in the solution as the source of Fe, so that an unknown proportion of the Cd (as well as of the other heavy metals) was present in chelated form. The amount of EDTA absorbed by plants from such systems is controversial, but it might have served here to transport some Cd from roots to tops.

The possibility of such high uptake of cadmium in practice is reinforced by Webber's work [65] in which CdO or $CdSO_4$ was added to pots of John Innes compost of pH 6.1 and radish, lettuce, and red beet were grown. All three crops were reduced in yield by the addition of 100 mg/kg Cd, at which level the content in the plant was of the order of 200 ppm, being higher with CdO than with $CdSO_4$. At higher levels the crops failed. While one must be cautious in extrapolating pot tests to the field, still this work is by far the most disturbing yet to appear. We are not told the c.e.c. of the compost, but it could hardly be less than 50 meq/100 g or 500 eq/million, and here we have 2 eq Cd/million of soil as already excessive, or 0.4% of c.e.c. at most. It might be argued that the normally antagonistic ions (Ca, Mn, Zn, etc.) are inactivated on the compost while the Cd is presented in the most reactive form, a solid of low but sufficient solubility. However, the harmful effect was observed on a second crop as well as the first, so time had been allowed to approach a kind of equilibrium.

3.6.3 Fate of Cd Applied in Superphosphate

Cadmium occurs as a trace metal in rock phosphate and hence enters into superphosphate. The Cd thus applied to soil in normal agriculture is much more soluble than native Cd and its history may be followed both by extracting the soil with normal HCl and by analyzing crops grown on the soil.

The superphosphate followed by Williams and David [22] in country near Canberra, Australia, averaged 40 ppm Cd. This Cd was found to be taken up by plants growing on a loam of pH 6 as readily as was that of added $CdCl_2$. Further, after varying amounts of superphosphate, from 1,000 to 4,500 kg/ha, had been added over 30 to 45 years, the Cd in the surface soil in excess over that in neighboring unfertilized soils, as extracted with normal HCl, came to 80% of the calculated addition in the fertilizer; there is good reason to believe that the remainder had passed below the 10 cm level rather than reverting to less soluble forms. The authors stress the geochemical analogy between Cd and Ca; both of these move downward much more easily than does added phosphate.

The various pasture plants growing on the soil topdressed over the years with superphosphate take up different amounts of Cd. The standard legume of the region, subterranean clover, is a collector and contained 0.3 and 0.4 ppm Cd where 2,500 kg/ha of superphosphate had been added, incorporating only 100 g/ha Cd. But the Cd in wheat grain remains low, since the wheat plant does not transport it readily to the tops and transfers only 15% of the total Cd in the tops to the grain. Australian wheat grain, in spite of the long history of superphosphate, typically contains only 0.02 ppm Cd.

3.7 UPTAKE AND TOLERANCE OF NICKEL

Most studies of excess Ni have been centered on soils formed on serpentine, for example, Crooke's work [8] with a soil containing 300 ppm Ni exchangeable with $ZnSO_4$, and Anderson and coworkers' where the uptake of Co and Cr was also measured [65]. Liming the soil has always greatly reduced the damage. However, the plant after liming continues to absorb high amounts of Ni, for example 80 to 100 ppm in oats. The lime is not merely raising the pH; one spectacular success occurred [66] where the pH was raised only from 5.7 to 6.5. The Ca thus provided is antagonistic to the Ni within the plant. Mn toxicity likewise is well known to be ameliorated by raising the Ca level within the plant. In an experiment adding $NiCl_2$ to soil [67] 500 ppm Ni was added to a soil of pH 6.4 and 21% organic matter without damaging the oat crop (say 2.5% of c.e.c.).

One pot experiment [29] has tested the addition of $NiSO_4$ to a neutral peat, with oats and soybeans being grown. Both crops were unaffected at 1,000 ppm and damaged at 2,000, at which level the plant content exceeded 50 ppm.

Little has been published about the tolerance of different species for Ni, except that the gramineae are found to be relatively tolerant. Ni seems to differ from the other heavy metals in being often more concentrated in seed than in straw.

3.8 UPTAKE AND TOLERANCE OF LEAD

Lead is strongly precipitated by soil (Section 2.4.8). Yet many plants take up as much as 30 ppm in their roots. Most plants retain this Pb almost entirely in the roots [68]. While we may generally be right to ignore the Pb in roots since it does not move into the tops, such movement was noted for sulfur-deficient ryegrass, which accumulated over 25 ppm in tops [9]. In other cases where such values as 30 ppm have been recorded in the tops, the plant has shown no ill effect. In another experiment [69], a soil with 21% organic matter was given 500 ppm Pb as $PbCl_2$, and the oat crop growing on it contained only 5 ppm in the straw and less than 1 ppm in grain. In general, if there is reason to worry over contanination of crops with lead, it should be over deposition from the air, not uptake by plants.

CHAPTER 4

CROPPING WITH SEWAGE WASTES CONTAINING HEAVY METALS

4.1 NATURE OF SEWAGE SLUDGE

There are many kinds of sewage wastes applied to land, including both raw liquid sewage, and liquid or solid products that have passed through various stages and kinds of microbial and chemical treatment. The more prolonged the microbial treatment, the more the reactive organic materials will have been decomposed and the more stable the residual solids will be.

When liquid and solid phases are eventually separated the heavy metals are present in far higher concentration in the solid than in the liquid phase. To a first degree of approximation the total weight of metal is distributed equally between solid and liquid, so if we take the ratio of liquid to final solid as 5,000:1, the concentration (as ppm) will be 5,000 times as high in the solid. (The ratio comes from the figures of 100 gallons of water and 100 dry sludge per cap. daily.) This attraction of the metal to the solid follows from its characteristics as negatively charged colloid, and introduces us to the fact that plants growing on mixtures of soil and sludge may absorb very little heavy metal, even if the total amount added in the sludge is impressive. The weight of 20 ha-cm of effluent (2,000 tons) is only 200 times that of a modest application of sludge (10 tons), so it would add 1/25 as much heavy metal. Discussion is reasonably concentrated therefore on the fate of heavy metals when applied in sludge.

Sewage may be treated through microbial decomposition to form "activated sewage sludge"; this may be further treated by prolonged anaerobic digestion at high temperature to form "digested sludge." Activated sewage sludge will further decompose rapidly, and lose one-third of its organic content during the next few months, while digested sludge decomposes at about the rate of one-sixth per annum. It is often described as "stabilized" since its most reactive components have disappeared. The active nitrogenous constituents too will depend on treatment, especially on aging, when the ammonium ion, a first-class source of nitrogen, slowly diminishes. Whatever the final proportion of ammonium, the organic product of anaerobic digestion is a good second-class source of soluble nitrogen, liberating its supply gradually so that as much as 120 tons of such sludge to a hectare may be needed to provide for a good corn crop, with the supply continuing for some years after application. It is assumed here that the interaction of heavy metals with sludges of the same pH but of otherwise different treatment is similar as soon as the most reactive fraction has decomposed. This seems probable and there is no evidence to the contrary.

Treatment may also include chemical additions for clarification and removal of phosphate, commonly either ferric or aluminum salts, any excess of which is precipitated as hydroxide at the high pH prevailing. Thus the sludge contains these inorganic hydroxides and phosphates as well as the original organic residues. (How much phosphate ends up thus combined with Fe and Al may be left an open question.)

The sludge contains various inorganic materials in addition: first, the industrial wastes which are the source of much of the heavy metals; second, miscellaneous grits and muds, which enter unavoidably as washings from streets.

All of these factors — different biological treatment, different chemical additives, different contamination with industrial wastes and grits and muds — play a part in the large differences in composition exhibited whenever analyses are collected from miscellaneous sources.

TABLE 4.1

Range and Median Values for Total Contents of Heavy Metals in 42 Sewage Sludges from Locations in England and Wales, Together with Typical Values for Soils, as Parts per Million in Dry Material*

Element	Sewage Sludge		Soil
	Range	Median	Typical
Ba	150-4,000	1,500	1,000
Cd	Tr-1,500	-	0.1
Cr	40-8,800	250	100
Cu	200-8,000	800	20
Fe	6,000-62,000	21,000	40,000
Mn	150-2,500	400	800
Ni	20-5,300	80	50
Pb	120-3,000	700	30
Zn	700-49,000	3,000	80

*From Ref. 70.

4.1.1 Total Content of Heavy Metals in Sludges

The heavy metal contents of a large number of sludges from various countries have been published, particularly from Sweden and Great Britain as well as the United States. A British tabulation [70] is given in Table 4.1: the general picture is similar to the American, and the median figures for the foreign metals may be compared with the geometric means for the United States calculated by Dean and Smith [71]. Table 4.1 also includes for comparison the two common heavy metals (Fe and Mn) and the omnipresent Ba, which is dealt with in Section 3.1. A median for Cd could not be derived in the British work since so many sludges had amounts too low to analyze; the American geometric mean was 61 ppm.

The first fact to emphasize about these figures is that they are highly variable and averages can be misleading. But Zn is almost always present in the highest amounts among the foreign metals and Cu is usually second, though Cr or Ni or Pb may predominate over Cu according to local industry. Another important feature is the distinction between residential and industrial sources (Table 4.2). With the former, only Zn and Cu are present in high amounts (though well below most industrial sludges); these two metals are used in water pipes as well as in other fittings. The other foreign metals may be introduced also into domestic sludge since drainage from roads adds products from car exhausts and tires.

Some of the industrial component can be controlled by local bodies, and many towns and cities in the United States have greatly reduced the heavy metal content of their sludges in recent years, so that the high figures quoted in Table 4.2 are no longer representative. There is a limit to this improvement, however. A recent analysis of the sources of heavy metals entering the waste-water system in New York [73] shows that electroplating (apart from nickel) is not responsible for high values, and that domestic sources and run-off from roads are responsible for two-thirds of the contribution of Cd, Cu, and Zn.

One must expect to find the heavy metals more concentrated in the product of a heated anaerobic treatment, since as much as one-third of the organic content disappears during this treatment while the metal remains. The fact that this difference does not demonstrate itself in some published lists serves to illustrate the wide and almost random range of the compositions.

Reports on the application of sludge may be given as so many dry tons per acre or hectare or as so many inches or centimeters of a suspension of a certain concentration, from which the dry ton-

TABLE 4.2

Components of (a) an Industrial Sludge* and (b) a Domestic Sludge**

	(a) Content in dry matter		(a) Content recalculated in terms of organic matter		(b) Content in dry matter		(b) Content recalculated in terms of organic matter	
	%	ppm	%	ppm	%	ppm	%	ppm
Calcium	5.1		11.2		3.7		5.9	
Phosphorus	3.5		7.8		1.3		2.1	
Nitrogen (organic)	1.5		3.3		(4.2)†		(6.7)†	
(inorganic, NH_4)	0.3							
Iron	4.0		8.9		1.0		1.6	
Cadmium		650		1,400		11		18
Chromium		5,000		11,000		—		—
Copper		2,900		6,400		1,100		1,800
Lead		2,200		4,900		440		700
Manganese		340		750		150		240
Nickel		500		1,100		30		50
Zinc		10,300		23,000		2,100		3,400
Loss on ignition	45		—		63		—	
pH	6.7		—		7.2		—	

* As used at Arcola. Source, Chicago.

** From Ref. 72.

† These figures are for total N and may contain a high proportion of NH_4-N.

nage may be calculated. Weights quoted throughout this book are in terms of dry tons; one needs the information on the heavy metals as commonly published as milligrams per kilogram or parts per million in order to know the weight of metal applied per hectare. But one also needs another piece of information that is less often supplied, namely the organic content and the nitrogen content of the sludge. The organic content may be no more than half the total dry weight, meaning that the load of the heavy metals on the organic matter is double what it appears to be. The nearest available measure of this organic content is the loss on ignition, which has been used in the calculations in Table 4.2. The use of this involves errors up and down, but mostly it exaggerates the true value because some of the loss on heating consists of water from inorganic components such as hydrated ferric oxides.

The organic content of the sludge may be roughly computed, as the organic content of soil sometimes is, by multiplying the organic N figure by 20. The figure for nitrogen is interesting apart from this calculation since it provides another practical measure of the burden of the heavy metals. The chief attraction of the heavy use of sludge for crops is that it provides a slow and steady release of ammonium and nitrate. If it supplies all the needs of a corn crop for nitrogen, then every ton harvested has involved the use of 18 kg N. The two sludges compared in Table 4.2 represent two extremes. The first, which is highly metalliferous and also aged, has a Zn:N ratio of 1:1.8 while the second, which comes from a residential district and is dominated by Zn and Cu, has a Zn:N ratio of 1:20. Thus if one arbitrarily decides that a total of 500 kg Zn may be tolerated in a hectare, this will have been accumulated after the harvesting of a bonus of 50 tons using the former sludge, or of 550 using the latter.

Table 4.2 includes also figures for P which call for comment. The phosphate is not only a rich reserve for plants, but it much exceeds the heavy metals (P has half the atomic weight of Zn) so is likely to offset at least any damage that they may do by antagonizing phosphate. Sulfur (only a small proportion of which is soluble sulfate) was not available for these two sludges but is commonly about 1%. This includes an unknown amount of sulfide. Sewage engineers have stressed the value of sulfide in lowering the concentration of heavy metals in solution at the works and so allowing bacterial reactions that might otherwise have been inhibited. We do not know how much sulfide is present in the final sludge, but Cu and Pb will combine and precipitate as sulfide before Zn or Ni.

A highly detailed analysis of an industrial sludge is reported by Peterson et al. [74] together with discussion of other sludges in relation to treatment.

4.1.2 Forms of Heavy Metals in Sludges

In dealing with soil, the first question one would ask about the analytical figure for any element is, "What form is it in?" The total amount of nitrogen in the topsoil of a hectare might be 4,000 kg, which might liberate anything from 80 to 250 kg in a year as nitrate, depending on how it has been farmed; or if it is a peaty sand it might liberate only 10 kg. So too the total amount of a trace element is hardly relevant, except very roughly. A soil might contain a silicate crystal with 1% copper. This copper would be reported in a total analysis, yet it is buried from the plant, and the only reason for considering the figure is that some of the copper must have weathered over the ages and come into circulation.

But the question has different implications for sludge. There will be no deeply buried atoms as in, say, a feldspar. Rather, one may consider the system as a mixture of individual ions and colloids starting out anew — so much organic material in sludge with its negative charges and chelating groups, so much sulfide, so much of the ions of copper and zinc and the rest. Perhaps some zinc is there as oxide, but this is not a means of removal since ZnO is an ideal zinc fertilizer, and as already noted, CdO is more damaging than $CdSO_4$ [64]. Even if some metals are there as sulfides, they are not thereby kept out of their regular cycles, since sulfides are microbially oxidized. For example, Steenbjerg and Boken [75] cured copper deficiency on the sandy soils of Jutland by adding finely ground bornite ($CuFeS_2$). Thus we can regard the bulk of the metals as (actually or potentially) adsorbed, adsorbed-chelated, or soluble-chelated in small amounts.

Little attempt has yet been made to separate the particles of sludge mechanically into their components, and when this is done some refinement may become possible on the above suggestion that total figures are far more valuable when quoted for sludge than for soil. Meanwhile we have two lines of work that are more refined. One, the extraction of sludge with citric-citrate buffers [76], shows that more than half the total Zn and Cu was extractable at pH 3, and almost half at pH 5. The other, the extraction with N/2 acetic acid [70], gave highly variable results for all the metals, with Zn the most soluble and Cr the least. The differences among the metals are those expected. The variability using this gentle reagent is also not surprising; the pH of the extracting solution must have varied greatly, for instance.

When this system is mixed with soil the reaction of the metals is now widened to include clay colloid and soil organic colloid, which will compete with the sludge. There seems to have been no substantial study of this competition. Here again we are in an obscure region. One would expect that the organic colloids of sludge and soil would be similar in holding power and buffering power. Yet most measurements of the c.e.c. of metalliferous sludge, whether using NH_4 or Ba as the replacing ion, indicate a value for its organic matter less than half that of soil organic matter. Now one can calculate that if Zn occupies a place permanently and cannot be ousted, then every 320 ppm of Zn added to a soil will decrease the c.e.c. by 1 meq/100 g, and conceivably some of the explanation lies there. At the same time, the holding power of sludge depends on pH as does that of soil; one of the worst effects on crops reported with a metalliferous sludge [77] happened when the pH of the sludge had fallen to 4.3, while a neutral sludge has been successfully used to *overcome* metal toxicity [78].

4.2 CROPPING WITH SEWAGE AND SLUDGE APPLIED AT HIGH RATES

It may surprise the newcomer to the subject that so much uncertainty surrounds a practice which is as old as this century — that is, the agricultural use of organic wastes which carry a burden of zinc and other metals. Yet the area concerned has been small, and the proportion of this treated area which has been heavily dosed with heavy metals is itself small. There have been a few warning voices, and a few reports of damage. Those that deserve serious attention are discussed below, as are corresponding favorable reports.

4.2.1 Unfavorable Evidence, Especially from Great Britain

The most solid pieces of unfavorable evidence come from Great Britain in accounts by members of the Agricultural Development and Advisory Service.

Webber [35] reports field experiments growing red beets, celery, and lettuce on a silt loam of pH between 6 and 7 treated with sludges which were chosen as being respectively high in zinc, copper, nickel, and chromium. (As he pointed out, metals do not occur singly in high concentrations in sludges, and there was more Zn than Ni in the "nickel" sludge, but this is not a serious fault of the experiments.) The results are difficult to summarize in tabular form, since sludges were used at different rates per hectare as well as at different metal concentrations. Most of those chosen for the experiment were near the maximum metal concentrations on record for sludges. (The purpose was to set up criteria for limits.) Much the lightest treatment consisted of two annual applications each of 31 ton/ha of sludge carrying, respectively, 4,000 ppm Zn (so totalling 250 kg/ha), 2,000 ppm Cu (125 kg/ha), 1,000 ppm Ni (62 kg/ha), and 1,100 ppm Cr. At these levels beet was somewhat damaged by the Zn but not by the other metals, while celery was not damaged by any metal. At all higher applications of metal per hectare the yield of beet was greatly reduced by Zn, Cu, and Ni; but celery was not decreased by Zn up to 1,000 kg/ha, by Cu to 500 kg/ha, by Ni to 250 kg/ha, while lettuce tolerated Cu to 250 kg/ha and Ni to 125 kg/ha. No adverse results from Cr were observed in this work, in keeping with general experience.

The above figure for initial damage to beet by a sludge with 4,000 ppm Zn corresponds to 12.5 meq/100 g of sludge. This probably exceeded 10% of the c.e.c. of the sludge but could not have reached 10% of the mixed sludge and soil.

These unfavorable results were obtained with high amounts of added metal, and one of the species used (red beet) is known to be especially sensitive to zinc. The contemporaneous report by Patterson [79] refers to several cases where total amounts of metal were not so high but where there was damage by zinc, to wheat as well as sugar-beet, and damage by nickel, to oats and potatoes. Patterson quotes his experience that damage is rarely due to a single element but comes from the combined effect of a number of elements. The term synergism is used where one element reinforces the toxicity of another.

At this point one should refer the reader to the summary by Chaney [80] where the theory as discussed here is covered in short space, and where much new information is supplied on the performance of various crops on soils with additions of heavy metals, especially Cd and Zn. Since the dominant note in his article is one of caution, it belongs to the present section of this book.

Without spending time on the predictably bad results of applying strongly acid sludge [77] (which liberated much Zn to solution) we may consider three long-term experiences of city sewage farms, one of which (Melbourne) is wholly favorable, another (Paris) is also favorable although it has been inaccurately quoted as the reverse, while the third (Berlin) is not favorable, though the evidence is incomplete.

4.2.2 The Heavy Metals in Three Old Sewage Farms

The sewage farms of the title are those of three capital cities: Paris, Berlin, and Melbourne. All of them are running concerns today and have been recipients of heavy metals throughout their careers, so that information about the state of these metals in soil and plant today should throw light on discussions in other countries. They have been irrigated with raw sewage that has had no more treatment than settling, by which much heavy metal has been removed but much still remains, as can be seen from the following analyses. At Paris and Berlin sewage is used to grow vegetables for human consumption; at Werribee (the Melbourne farm) it grows pasture for beef cattle and sheep.

Paris Farms

The soil is a sandy loam of pH 7.0 measured in KCl — that is, it is definitely alkaline — and contains a little free $CaCO_3$. It is formed on the Seine alluvium.

The published information about heavy metals in the soil at Paris comes from two sources. First, Rohde [81] whose work is best known to English readers through an abridged and unsatisfactory translation [82]; second, a French group from whom the fullest report is by Trocmé et al. [83] on manganese deficiency in vegetables, especially in leeks, spinach, and potatoes. From these sources one can confidently summarize the situation.

Rohde uses the prescientific term "exhaustion" (Rieselmüdigkeit) for the state of the soil at both Paris and Berlin after copper and zinc have accumulated; the evidence for this exhaustion is that plants make poor growth and are chlorotic. The French authors report that manganese deficiency had occurred on scattered areas over 25 years before their paper appeared. This disease has an alarming appearance and may wipe out a crop, and some areas had been abandoned. In more recent years the disease has been completely overcome by frequent spraying with $MnSO_4$ solution. Rohde knew that this treatment was beneficial but did not recognize that the conquest of the trouble makes nonsense of the word "exhaustion."

Trocmé et al. had correctly identified the trouble but were baffled in trying to interpret it in terms of manganese alone. Like Rohde, they found that the affected sites contained 50 to 100% more organic matter than the healthy sites (5 to 8% against 2 to 4%); they were in slight depressions where the water lay longer. Rohde knew about the manganese deficiency, but it did not occur to him that this could be the only trouble caused by heavy metals in the sewage. He blames both copper and zinc, but his extractions of soils with boiling water under reflux do not support the case against copper. Typical figures for affected sites against healthy sites are 5.4 ppm against 1.9 ppm for zinc and 11.2 against 8.5 for copper — these copper figures, while both very high, are not very different. While both elements are antagonistic to manganese, the antagonism of zinc is more widely known, and will be followed here while leaving open the possible effect of copper. In the author's experience, "gray speck" (manganese deficiency) has occurred in oats grown under bird-proof wire, when the acid rain of a city has dissolved the zinc coating from the wire and sprayed the plants below with dilute zinc sulfate, this antagonistic effect occurring even on a soil of pH below 6.

The sites with more organic matter had received more sewage and more zinc, which amounted to roughly 1.2% of the organic matter. The total manganese was no higher or was even lower on the affected sites, so that the ratio of active Zn to active Mn was probably much higher on the affected sites. Trocmé et al. quote the raw irrigating water as containing 0.05 ppm Mn and 0.10 ppm Zn, while the drainage contained 0.10 ppm Mn and 0.015 ppm Zn — that is, the Mn was being steadily impoverished by waterlogging and leaching, while the Zn steadily accumulated. We do not know the figures for the soluble Mn and Zn in the root zone, and without them the situation is puzzling. Yet there is no doubt about the Mn deficiency, and the case for antagonism is supported by their figures in Table 4.3, though they do not say so themselves. It appears that the zinc has done no further damage than to antagonize the manganese — and perhaps no more should be expected since the degree of saturation of organic matter with zinc has remained constant in both good and bad sites. Zinc can do other damage to plants, but perhaps this does not easily happen where phosphate is so amply supplied as here. The stunting that has elsewhere been reported with zinc has been attributed to its antagonism to phosphate. However, the soil at Paris, while it has only 7% clay, is calcareous and this would counter any further damage by zinc, in spite of the high figure of 0.1% Zn extracted by the not very drastic acid (Table 4.4).

TABLE 4.3

Analytical Figures for Leeks, Healthy and Unhealthy, and for Corresponding Soil at Paris*

	Leeks, tops (dry matter)				
	%		ppm		Soil, %
Type	N	P	Mn	Zn	N
Healthy	2.3	0.19	15	45	0.17
Unhealthy	3.8	0.43	9	110	0.52

*From Ref. 83.

TABLE 4.4

Mean Values for Extracts of Soils on Two Sewage Farms*

		ppm dissolved boiling N HCl		ppm dissolved boiling water	
Place	Type	Cu	Zn	Cu	Zn
Berlin	Healthy	118	197	8.7	6.5
	chlorotic	508	609	20.1	19.1
Paris	Healthy	132	386	8.5	3.4
	chlorotic	292	1,032	11.2	10.5

*From Refs. 81, 82.

Berlin Farm

Rohde's account [81,82] of the trouble at Berlin may be briefly mentioned, though the lack of further information makes it difficult to interpret. His figures for the "total" Cu and Zn dissolved by boiling normal HCl are given in Table 4.4. The crops with which he worked were mustard, cabbage, and maize. He is sure that the chlorosis of each of these was not due to manganese deficiency, and he is inclined to blame copper more than zinc. His extractions of soil with boiling water under reflux give remarkably high values (Table 4.4). He notes that liming the soil reduces the trouble, as does the drastic treatment of roasting, (temperature not mentioned), which greatly reduces the water-soluble Cu and Zn. Evidently he blames especially the soluble chelates formed by both metals for the troubles. His analyses throughout are of soils, not of plants.

Table 4.5 gives supplementary information including subsoils and showing the concentrating of metals in the surface as well as the high phosphate. (Note that a different extracting acid is used here.)

The soil pH in KCl averages 5.6; it is on the acid side, though only moderately so, but is very different from that of Paris. The soil is described as sand. As at Paris, there is about twice as much organic matter in soils with chlorotic as with healthy plants (loss on ignition 6.3 and 2.7% respectively).

Certainly this report must be counted as unfavorable to the use of city sewage on the land, though the picture is obscure.

Melbourne's Farm at Werribee

The Melbourne and Metropolitan Board of Works has a farm at Werribee which has served the city of Melbourne since 1893. The liquid raw sewage is used to irrigate the land. The sludge has not been applied to the land, so the heavy metals have not reached the totals found elsewhere; still they are high enough to be of interest to the present account. The area receiving sewage is 5,600 ha, which serves about two million people. (The area irrigated has increased with the growth of the city.)

TABLE 4.5

Parts per Million Phosphorus, Copper, and Zinc Extracted from Berlin Soils by Boiling Nitric Acid Described as "1:2"*

Type	Depth cm	P	Cu	Zn
	0-20	2,700	350	450
Irrigated,	30-40	2,100	60	130
chlorotic plants	60-70	2,300	30	90
	0-20	2,600	90	160
Irrigated,	30-40	2,200	30	70
healthy plants	60-70	2,100	20	60
Unirrigated healthy plants	0-20	2,200	20	80

*From Refs. 81,82.

The land under irrigation is flat to gently sloping and is part of the alluvial plain of the Werribee River near its outlet to Port Phillip Bay. The soil is silty clay loam to clay with a saline subsoil at 75 cm high in exchangeable sodium. During the earlier years of the farm the soil was broken up with tines to a depth of 75 cm, with the hope of thereby making it more permeable. The infiltration averages 2 cm a day, and is probably not different from its original figure. The soil averages 40% of clay below 2 μm. The main feature of the present-day profile is the consequence of irrigation; namely a highly organic surface 2 to 3 cm with substantial organic nitrogen in the top 18 cm, together with the varying pattern of deposition of the elements brought in by the sewage, as here set out. The organic carbon in the top 2.5 cm reaches 17% in three of the six samples reported. The pH of the surface has an average of 6 but varies from place to place, being lower in the sites with a longer history of irrigation.

The irrigation of 110 cm, all of which either infiltrates or evaporates, is carried out during the six warmer months of the year when the mean air temperature is above 14°C, reaching a mean of 20°C in the hottest months, when evaporation can be very high. "Grass filtration" is carried out during the cooler months, whereby sewage is run over other portions of the farm without much infiltration. The yearly rainfall averages 48 cm, which is evenly spread over the 12 months.

The land has been continuously under pasture since 1914, and is grazed by 13,000 beef cattle together with some sheep. The plant species differ with situation. Rye grass occupies well-drained sites, while the lower land on each run is wet for longer periods after irrigation and carries other species including docks and barley grass; water couch occurs in the wettest areas. The various pasture species may differ in their uptake of heavy metals, but no survey of this sort has been made.

The soil in the irrigated area was sampled at six different sites in June, 1972 and a neighboring unirrigated soil (i.e., never treated with sewage) was sampled as a control. All soils were taken at three levels, namely 0 to 2.5, 2.5 to 18, 25 to 45 cm. All samples were analyzed for various elements, some total and some by extraction with N/10 HCl. The more important results are collected in Tables 4.6 and 4.7 [6]. The most striking figures in Table 4.6 are those for Zn which in this mobile form is highly concentrated in the surface, especially in the uppermost (organic) 2.5 cm, but which has also moved considerably below 18 cm; the individual samples with the highest accumulation in the top 2.5 cm (not shown in this table) were also those that showed this downward movement most clearly. The same pattern, though with only 1% of the amount, is shown by Cd, and a similar pattern, also on a smaller scale, by Ni. While Pb also is concentrated in the uppermost 18 cm, it appears to be less so in the organic layer, which disagrees with most pedological experience; but the samples here are too variable for a firm conclusion. The very small addition of mobile Cu should be set beside the total figure in Table 4.6; perhaps a chelator would be a better extracting agent for mobile Cu than the dilute HCl, but this was not tried. Comparison of Tables 4.6 and 4.7 shows that about two-thirds of the total Zn added during this century is still extractable by N/10

TABLE 4.6

Heavy Metals Extracted from Werribee Soils by Cold N/10 HCl (1:5) Shaken for 18 Hours*

		ppm of air-dry soil				
Type	Depth, cm	Cd	Cu	Ni	Pb	Zn
Irrigated	0-2.5	1.8	2.0	13.0	6.2	210
	2.5-18	0.6	4.1	4.8	11.1	70
	25-45	0.2	2.9	4.6	1.0	17
Unirrigated	0-2.5	0.2	1.1	1.9	5.6	16
	2.5-18	Tr	0.8	1.0	2.2	2
	25-45	Tr	2.2	2.9	1.1	1

*Mean of six sites for irrigated; one site unirrigated.

TABLE 4.7

Total Heavy Metals in Werribee Soils*

		ppm of air-dry soil		
Type	Depth, cm	Cu	Ni	Zn
Irrigated	0-2.5	82	45	340
	2.5-18	60	45	143
	25-45	55	60	100
Unirrigated	0-2.5	23	30	70
	2.5-18	21	30	60
	25-45	47	60	85

* Mean of six sites for irrigated; one site unirrigated.

HCl, and Ni is somewhat similar though the figures are not exact enough for a firm statement to be made. Clearly a great deal of Cu has been fixed in the surface soil.

The metals shown in these tables are those of most interest for our main topic. Co and Cr were also determined in the HCl extract and show surface increases of only 2 ppm, though far more Cr than this has been added.

Phosphorus has accumulated in large quantities. One site to which the heaviest amount of sewage had been applied was sampled in 1958 [1], and showed an additional 3,200 ppm P in the surface 10 cm, one-third of which was in the organic form.

A few figures for plant material are collected in Table 4.8, representing means of four irrigated sites compared with one unirrigated. The plants were taken in June, when grasses are limited as much by low soluble nitrogen as by cold, mean temperature being $10^{o}C$. The higher fertility of the irrigated land in N and P is shown as expected. The Zn and Cu contents on the irrigated land are double those of the unirrigated, but are far below any dangerous level. The highest concentration of Zn in plants, namely 150 ppm, occurred on the soil with the highest acid-soluble Zn, namely 438 ppm. This is the main interesting difference. The higher value for Mn in the unirrigated plants is unimportant; not only were the species different, but the site had a low pH which would lead to high Mn in plants.

No trouble associated with heavy metals in plants has been reported on the metropolitan farm. The only heavy-metal trouble with the grazing animals has been a minor deficiency of copper, confirmed by liver analysis. The reason for this is not yet understood.

While systematic analytical figures for the metals in raw sewage and in drains have not been published, Table 4.9 summarizes averages obtained through the year 1974, as found by the staff of Melbourne and Metropolitan Board of Works.

TABLE 4.8

Composition of Plant Material Growing on Irrigated and Unirrigated Land at Werribee (June, 1972)

	%, oven-dry weight				ppm, oven-dry weight				
Type	N	P	Ca	K	Cd	Cu	Mn	Ni	Zn
Irrigated	3.8	0.57	0.30	3.0	0.9	14	51	6	104
Unirrigated	1.8	0.29	0.33	1.9	0.8	6	149	3	50

TABLE 4.9

Parts per Million (mg/liter) of Heavy Metals in Solution at Werribee, 1974

Type	Cd	Cr	Cu	Ni	Pb	Zn
Raw sewage	0.02	0.42	0.31	0.21	0.12	1.1
Drains	0.005	0.1	0.04	0.06	0.03	0.08

4.2.3 Favorable Evidence from Illinois

While several local reports on the agricultural use of sewage sludge have appeared in publications or semipublications, special attention is given here to reports from Illinois, from which the results of both published and hitherto unpublished work are summarized. These provide the most substantial evidence of the application of metalliferous sludge to the land without ill effects. They include the use of especially heavy amounts of sludge with high concentrations of heavy metals, together with monitoring of drains. Such heavy applications, which are made in 1:10 suspensions in water, are only possible where land is almost flat.

1. Farmland at Arcola

The site at Arcola (Soil Enrichment Materials Corporation) is typical of the corn belt of Illinois. The land is flat to gently sloping, the soil a dark clay loam (Drummer series) with 4.5% organic matter and pH 6.0 with clay subsoil of fair permeability. The sludge, an anaerobically digested product of composition given in Table 4.2, was applied in 1970 and 1971 at rates varying over different parcels of land, ranging from 0 (in areas set aside as controls) to as much as 225 dry tons/ha, the bulk of the land receiving 55 dry tons/ha; the sludge was plowed in to the top 18 cm of soil. The various treatments comprised about 160 ha.

The field corn and soybeans, standard varieties for the district, were sown in spring 1972 and 1973 and 1974. They grew well at all rates of application and showed no sign of excess or deficiency of any nutrient. The figures quoted here are for 1972.

Contents of Heavy Metals in Crops: The results of analyses for total heavy metals in corn leaves (sampled in summer) and harvested grain are collected in Table 4.10. The values for the metals growing with sludge come from 10 samplings with different rates; but since the uptake of metals did not increase with increasing applications of sludge, all that is tabulated is the range. For five of the seven heavy metals tested (Cr, Cu, Hg, Ni, Pb) sludge did not affect the uptake at all. For the other two (Cd, Zn) sludge led to a fivefold increase in leaf content, though only Zn of these two has a higher content in grain. This result is in keeping with both theory and practice which show that Cd and Zn are the most soluble of the heavy metals in soils. Apart from the excessive uptake of Cd in corn leaves, all these figures fall in the common range reported in the reference books.

TABLE 4.10

Parts per Million of Heavy Metals in Dry Matter of Crop at Arcola (1972)

Type	With (+) or without sludge (-)	Cd	Cr	Cu	Hg*	Ni	Pb	Zn
Corn leaf	+	10-15	1.5-2.5	12-16	15-25	2-4	4-9	100-250
	-	1-2	2.0	15	20-23	2-4	5-7	25-30
Corn grain	+	0.1-0.3	0.5	5-7	1-3	1.5-3	0.2-0.8	20-35
	-	0.1	0.5	5-6	2-4	1.5-2	0.2-1.5	10-20
Soybean leaf	+	1-5	0.5-1	17	30	8-14	4	80-160
	-	0.5	0.5	15	25-60	8	4	40
Soybean grain	+	1-2	0.5-0.7	15-20	2-3	10-15	2	50-110
	-	0.3-0.6	0.5-1.3	15	1.5-3	2-6	2	45

*Parts per billion.

Soybeans also were analyzed, but information is less than for corn; the results mostly follow those for corn, with increase being confined to Zn and Cd. The Cd in the seed, however, is higher, with values just exceeding 1 ppm in two successive years.

The steady figure for uptake of heavy metal with increasing quantities of sludge in 1972, especially when these quantities were high, calls for comment. It appears that the sludge itself carried the main burden of withholding the metal from plants, so that in the first year the treated soil was merely a diluent of the sludge. This situation is opposite to that of the common use of a fertilizer such as phosphate, which is added in small amounts to an excess of soil which strongly reacts with it, so that one expects uptake to increase with increasing fertilizer. This explanation is supported by the figures for 1974, when the content of Cd in both corn and soybean increased with higher applications of sludge, indicating that the protection was passing from the sludge to the soil. In this year one sample of corn grain on a heavily sludged area reached 1 ppm Cd.

Metals in Drainage: The tile drains and wells of the treated area and wells upstream were repeatedly tested for the heavy metals (besides soluble nitrogen, etc.). The representative figures where sludge had been applied were much less than the state standard for waters; typical levels were 0.02 mg/liter for Cd, 0.02 mg/liter for Cu, 0.06 mg/liter for Pb, 0.0003 mg/liter for Hg, and 0.15 mg/liter for Zn. An occasional higher value was observed, notably for Hg. If sludge had been responsible for a high value, this would be bound to be steady and not erratic; and, in fact, the odd high values were found on the same day outside and upstream from the sludged land. The most obvious reason for such an occurrence is the application of a mercurial fungicide on the land upstream.

2. Plot Tests at Joliet

These tests [84] were done on 75 m^2 replicated plots, suspended sludge being added in the furrows between rows of corn, and the same plots being treated continuously for 4 years. The sludge was produced from the heated anaerobic digester of Chicago, and the added load of heavy metals after 160 dry tons/ha had been spread may be seen in Table 4.11. The soil used, Blount silt loam, was first left in its acid state, but after the pH in some sludge plots had

TABLE 4.11

Amount of Heavy Metals in Surface 15 cm of Soil, 3 Years after First Application of Sludge, with Total 160 tons/ha Added*

	ppm oven-dry soil					
	Cd	Cr	Cu	Ni	Pb	Zn
Untreated soil, total element	1.1	29	19	23	31	72
Additional after treatment, total element	7.4	57	33	5	29	188

*From Ref. 84.

fallen below 5, limestone was applied to restore the pH to the control value (5.2). In spite of the acidity, which was deliberately incurred, all the treated crops were increased in yield over controls (which were given regular NPK fertilizer) and they showed no damage from the heavy metals. The sludge differed from that used at Arcola in being very high in ammonium, 1,550 kg NH_4-N/ha being so added each year.

As at Arcola, the uptake of Cr, Cu, Hg, Ni, and Pb was unaffected by sludge (Table 4.12), but that of Cd and Zn was increased, again with smaller increases in grain than in leaf, especially with Cd. Unlike Arcola, the uptake of both Cd and Zn increased linearly with application of sludge (only the maximum application is recorded in the table). This difference, implying greater solubility, is probably related to the much greater acidity of the soil-sludge mixture here, and is in keeping with the leaching of heavy metals which is revealed in the authors' Table 9. This result disagrees with the

TABLE 4.12

Parts per Million of Metal in Dry Matter of Crop, 1970, With and Without Addition of 160 tons/ha of Dry Sludge Spread Over 3 Years*

Type	With (+) or without (-) sludge	Cd	Cr	Cu	Hg	Ni	Pb	Zn
Corn leaf	+	11.6	4.5	8.7	0.04	4.3	6.3	212
	-	3.3	4.1	8.9	0.03	2.8	7.1	58
Corn grain	+	1.0	0.4	5.6	0.004	3.1	0.03	152
	-	0.3	0.3	5.2	0.005	2.3	0.03	89

*From Ref. 84.

conclusion reached above (Section 2.3.8) that a crop will show damage before heavy metals move substantially into drainage water; and is at present difficult to interpret. So the results here are not altogether favorable, but they exemplify good growth with a highly metalliferous sludge even on a soil of low pH.

Perhaps one should mention here an opinion that has been circulated in connection with this work, namely, that toxicity from excess phosphate is a serious risk in adding sludge to land. If this opinion were correct it would make nonsense of most of the present book. The evidence in favor of the belief in toxic phosphate is that a chlorosis of soybeans was observed after a heavy sludging. It sounds like Zn excess causing Mn deficiency, as happened at Paris, and until more is known this explanation should be sufficient.

3. Other Results

Other results are recorded by Peterson et al. [85] where sludge from Chicago of high metal content was successfully used in amounts of the order of 330 ton/ha in establishing growth of corn and of grass on waste land, in all cases without symptoms of toxicity. (It should be noted, however, that the figures for "cation exchange capacity" in their Tables 2 and 3 are not of c.e.c. but are merely the sum of exchangeable Ca, Mg, K, and Na.)

The favorable experiences may be set beside the earlier findings that where Zn was added without sludge it damaged plants when present to the order of 5% of c.e.c. at pH 6 and 20% at pH 7, and Webber's experiment with sludge [35] is in keeping with this. The Arcola results show that Zn present as 4 meq/100 g did no harm and did not accumulate in excessive amounts in corn, and here it exceeds 10% of c.e.c. A similar sludge applied at Ottawa, Illinois [74] at rates with the heavy metals certainly exceeding 20% of c.e.c. was similarly harmless and only beneficial; the pH of the soil-sludge mixture here was over 8.

Another study of the use of sludge from a residential area may be quoted here [86], since while similar encouraging results must have been obtained on numerous occasions in many countries, such detailed monitoring of the heavy metals in soils, crops, and drainage water as here carried out is still rare. The sludge was obtained from anaerobic digestion at Hanover Park, in the Chicago area. It contained (on an average) 44% volatile matter, 4.5% total N, and heavy metal contents (in parts per million) 50 Cd, 600 Cu, 250 Ni, 700 Zn. The soil was a silty clay loam of poor natural drainage, with pH 7.7 and c.e.c. 33 meq/100 g. The sludge was applied over 6 years amounting to 203 ton/ha and corn was grown continuously with grain yield averaging 5.5 ton/ha. During the 6 years the soil pH fell by 0.5.

The additional Zn added in the sludge over the years was 140 kg/ha, something of the order of 60 ppm in the soil, yet the amounts extracted from the soil by N/10 HCl do not reveal these additions; there is more variation from year to year than between treatments. The Zn content of leaves has almost doubled, but remains in the normal range below 100 ppm; the Zn content of grain is identical with that of controls, about 25 ppm. The additional Cd also is not extracted from the soil by N/10 HCl and does not reveal itself in any plant analysis. In keeping with these results, the drainage water was continually tested for heavy metals, and the values decreased to about 0.1 mg/liter for both Cu and Zn in the later years of the experiment.

4.2.4 Formulas for Limiting Use of Metalliferous Sludge

In this field where so much is still obscure and controversial, advisors and legislators have tried to draw lines dividing safe from dangerous applications of sludge. We will discuss here such lines in terms of damage to sensitive crops, and leave to a later section the risk of accumulating toxic amounts of a metal without necessarily decreasing the yield.

A formula for a dividing line between safe and dangerous applications of sludge was suggested by Webber [35] and set out by Chumbley [87]. One component in it, the "zinc equivalent," must first be explained.

The traditional chemical term "equivalent" used for Zn appearing in compounds like ZnO or $ZnCl_2$ means "half a gram-atom," or 32.7 g. But this special usage here introduced is quite different, and expresses the summed toxic effect of Cu and Ni when present together with Zn. Starting from the statement that Cu is twice as toxic to plants as the same weight of Zn, and Ni is eight times as toxic, a formula is arrived at that when all three metals are present together their total effect is additive, with these same weightings; so with A ppm Zn, B ppm Cu, C ppm Ni, the "Zn equivalent" of this sludge is $A + 2B + 8C$.

This formula is an invention made for the sake of prudence; it states that we have no solid information on the combined toxicity; therefore, we should assume the worst.

The first statement concerning relative toxicity might be accepted more readily than the second statement concerning additivity.

This is unknown as regards zinc plus nickel, though it might be true; but it is unlikely as regards zinc plus copper, which are often antagonistic.

Proposed Limit

The limit, as suggested by Webber and incorporated in an advisory paper by Chumbley, is an addition of 250 ppm of zinc equivalent if the pH is 6.5. The warning is given that a lower pH will lead to trouble. Transformed into degrees of saturation of c.e.c., this means that a soil of c.e.c. 16 meq/100 g could tolerate 5% of saturation with heavy metal without damage at pH 6.5. A later statement from the Environmental Protection Agency of the United States simultaneously doubles this allowance to 10% and makes the transformation explicit in terms of c.e.c. and not of total soil, so that we are no longer being expected to apply the same formula to a clay as to a sand [88].

This British formula was intended to apply equally to a single heavy application and to the same total application spread over 30 years. Where sludge is continuously applied, two opposing effects are at work over the years. On the favorable side, some of the heavy metal reverts to a form where it can be safely forgotten (a constant theme in this book, but one not mentioned explicitly in the British work). On the unfavorable side, organic matter oxidizes away (cf. Section 4.6.1) and at the best its protective effect cannot keep pace with the addition of metal. The only (indirect) reference to these two effects, both of which are obscure, is Webber's suggestion that the soil be extracted with half-normal acetic acid before the sludge is added, and the metal in this extract allowed for in making the calculation.

It is easy to find examples where the earlier British formula is far too cautious. Thus in the Arcola farm the heaviest application of sludge added 3,200 kg/ha of Zn, which is about six times the original proposed allowance in terms of Zn alone and 12 times the limit in terms of the zinc equivalent, and not only was no damage done but the grain of the crop contained normal amounts of Zn. But when the more liberal limit suggested by EPA is applied, namely 10% of c.e.c., then inserting the measured c.e.c. of 32 meq/100 g makes the successful application about 50% higher than the proposed limit without allowing for Cu and Ni, though still three times the proposed limit after incorporating Cu and Ni into the formula.

A major theme earlier in this book has been the steep dependence of adsorption on pH, with the suggestion (Section 2.5; Table I) that the critical figure for degree of saturation might well be 5% of c.e.c. at pH 6.0, 10% at pH 6.5, and 20% at pH 7.0. There are difficulties, however, in incorporating pH into a formula, a property so variable in time as well as space.

A bibliographic article by Baker and Chesnin [89], which gives much space to the impact of heavy metals on soils, accepts the EPA formula and concentrates on how to monitor it. The theoretical approach in this article differs greatly from that adopted here. First, it does not stress pH and does not deal with what is here called "reversion." Second, while emphasizing the role of organic matter as here, it depends on the "hydrous oxides" Fe_2O_3 and Al_2O_3 and MnO_2 as the inorganic fraction that adsorbs the heavy metals, with an implied theory (which is not discussed) that the major cations Ca and Mg take charge of the negative sites on clay which constitute the bulk of the c.e.c., while Zn and its associates take charge of the relatively few negative sites on the hydrous oxides. The question why the legal limit should be set by the c.e.c., namely by the clay which has only a broad relation to the hydrous oxides, is not discussed.

4.3 CROPPING WITH SLUDGE APPLIED AT LOW RATES: SLUDGE CONSIDERED AS SOURCE OF PHOSPHATE

The effects of heavy metals in sewage or sludge have been first discussed in terms of heavy treatments, whether continuous over many years as with sewage farms or in single applications as just discussed. Such treatments allow us to see the most unfavorable possibilities, and if plants or animals come to no harm at such levels, we may feel reassured at levels one-fiftieth as large.

The purpose of disposing sewage onto land could be merely to get rid of a nuisance. It could also, however, be aimed at saving a scarce resource, whether water, nitrogen, or phosphorus; and the contrast next to be considered depends on the choice of N or P as the valuable element to be saved. The treatments so far quoted have aimed at making the most of N — adding a slow-acting nitrogenous fertilizer which would continue to liberate a steady supply of ionic N for 5 years or more. But this involves adding P at a rate far higher than in normal agriculture, a typical figure in sludge being 2%. An alternative use of sludge would be as a source of P, so restoring that valuable element into circulation, together incidentally with other elements, notably S. This abandons the supply of N (which must be fulfilled from other sources) and loses the good physical effect of the organic content of the heavy treatment; but the burden of heavy metal is now cut to a small fraction of what was earlier considered.

If sludge is used for its P, a suitable application will now be from 1 to 1.5 ton/ha, (supplying 20 to 30 kg P). The application of heavy metal is now 1% of what was earlier considered. It will be 100 times better held by the soil colloids than before, and as well opposed by the added phosphate as before. Such a policy, if accepted by farmers, would clearly postpone any "day of reckoning" for many decades. While it is not incumbent on us to plan for a remote future with its possibly improved compositions of sludges as well as other unknowns, it is interesting to consider whether the new diminished risk still adds up over the decades. Two opposing trends are at work. On the one hand, the organic matter of the sludge disappears completely so that the protection against the heavy metal by organic matter settles down at that effected by the equilibrium figure of the soil's own organic matter. On the other hand, the metals revert to less active forms. There is no help from theory here, and perhaps decisions about safe total amounts of a given sludge to be added must rely on similar practical experiences to those already set out.

4.4 HEAVY METALS IN IRRIGATION WATER FROM SECONDARY TREATMENT

The effluent from sewage treatment may be valued for its content of nitrogen and phosphorus, besides supplying water at a convenient time. As with sludge, there is a question whether there is a price to be paid in heavy metals, even though the total amounts concerned are much less (and they are also less than in the sewage farms using untreated effluent).

While as a first approximation the total metal of the sewage is equally distributed between solid and liquid (Section 4.1), the metals vary in their distribution, with, for example, Zn being more retained in the solid and Ni and Cu remaining in the liquid by virtue of their soluble chelates. When effluents from different works are arranged in ascending order of heavy metals in solution, the great majority of them [90, 91] have less than 0.5 mg/liter of the metals of most concern to us (Cu, Zn, Ni, Pb). But since the exceptions to this statement include some large systems, the above figure will be used here for illustration. Cd is present in far smaller amounts, being often below the limit of detection and commonly below 0.01 mg/liter.

An element present in solution at 0.5 mg/liter and applied in irrigation at 150 cm annually would add 7.5 kg/ha in a year, whereas we have been considering doses up to 50 times as much in sludge, all added at once. The single addition in 1 year of irrigation, while perhaps twice what has been discussed in the preceding section, is still very small. If we accept the figure (Table I) that a soil of pH 6.0 might carry a heavy metal up to 5% of its c.e.c., without damage, and if its c.e.c. is 15 meq/100 g, then 5% of this would mean 480 kg Zn/ha-15 cm, to set beside the above figure of 7.5 kg annually. That is, such a soil would take the heavy metal for over 60 years before reaching a critical level. The situation would be four times as good at a pH of 7 as at 6, and again over twice as good for a soil with a high c.e.c. such as Arcola.

Trouble could arise with effluent only if a soil were strongly acid or if a sandy soil were chosen for irrigation, with little c.e.c.

of its own, and therefore leaving the organic matter derived from stubble and roots to give protection. In a hot climate with open cultivation there would be little such accumulation of organic matter. But apart from these extreme cases the danger is very small. And with effluent irrigation, as with sludge, the high application of phosphate has to be set against the effect of heavy metals.

Two cases of sewage irrigation continuing successfully through this century have already been quoted. In both places heavy amounts of zinc and copper have accumulated without damage. In one of them (Werribee) the soil is high in clay, the crop is grass (which may be tolerant), and much organic matter has accumulated. In the other (Paris) the soil is sandy but is slightly calcareous, and again some organic matter has accumulated. The crops at Paris (sundry vegetables) are not tolerant to heavy metals; perhaps the high combining power of organic matter at this high pH is a sufficient reason for continued success. But the main principle must be the same as already discussed (Section 4.2.4), namely that colloids will protect against the metal up to a certain degree of saturation.

Two differences between the two kinds of application — heavy sludge and annual effluent — should be mentioned. With small annual application of heavy metal continuing for decades one might hope for reversion; yet if this has happened at Werribee the analyses for Zn do not indicate it, though those for Cu do.

4.5 ACCUMULATION OF METALS IN FOOD CROPS

Some of the warnings over the use of metalliferous sludges have concerned not the possibility of damaging the crops but rather the accumulation of the metal in food, as, for example, the article by Berrow and Webber [70]. In fact, some of the better known reports of contamination of food by heavy metals (Warren et al. [92], Purves [93]) concern not the application of sewage sludge but aerial contamination and the use of coal ash and municipal compost as fertilizer in gardens. Even then, Purves's figures might be quoted for showing how little the heavy metal increases in plants even after large increases in soil. Each metal should be considered separately here. There is no cause for alarm at an increase in our Zn intake, which is generally deficient. On the other hand, the element most guilty of aerial contamination is lead, which is a serious threat but does not enter foods through the root. Without doubt, the metal of greatest concern in food is cadmium, which as discussed above (Section 3.6) can remain mobile in soils. Cd contents of sludged crops are included in some of the preceding sections; here we shall consider two Swedish studies [94,95] which centered on the uptake of Cd by wheat and rape from sludged soil in pots, and which have been considered alarming by some commentators. In both studies the soil was a loamy sand with 2.8% organic content and pH 4.8, which was adjusted over a range of pH by adding CaO. The sludge contained 10 ppm Cd and was applied at rates up to 175 ton/ha. At the time of harvesting the rape, 53 days after sowing, one-third of all added Cd was still extractable with M ammonium acetate at pH 4.8 — perhaps the most serious result of the experiment, though not surprising, and in keeping with the results of Williams and David (Section 3.6.3).

The concentration of Cd in the plants was decreased by the liming, as expected [94,95]. The highest level of Cd found in the wheat grain, adding 58 ton/ha sludge at pH 5.3, was only 0.26 ppm — and this with a soil freshly mixed with sludge and too sandy and too acid for good management with sludge. The rape, at 175 ton/ha sludge and pH 6.0, contained 0.6 ppm Cd. The figures do not give cause for alarm.

At this low end of the scale one should refer again to the use of Australian superphosphate containing 40 ppm Cd; this at 10% P is analogous to a sludge containing 10 ppm Cd and 2.5% P, such as just considered. During all this century, when this superphosphate has been used for growing wheat and since 1930 growing pasture for dairying and meat, 10 million tons of P (with its accompanying Cd) has been applied to the land, and no single case of damage by Cd to plant or animal or man on normal agricultural land has been found.

Above this level of Cd content in sludge there is no clear indication of where to draw a line. The old Chicago sludge (Table 4.2) with 50 times as much Cd as the Swedish, did not lead to a dangerous level of Cd in corn grain; the seed of soybean grown with the same sludge, however, reached or exceeded 1 ppm in the seed, and other crops might accumulate more Cd in their edible parts than does soybean seed.

We are on uncertain ground, therefore, in dealing with a sludge of the order of 100 ppm Cd, which might be with us for a few years. The addition of such a sludge at 25 ton/ha makes up 1 ppm of Cd in the surface soil, not only more than the likely native content, but more reactive. So long as the product is grain and is fed to livestock the situation is safe. But there remains a substantial region where analyses of leafy crops will be needed before one can feel assured.

4.6 MANAGEMENT

The debate over the risk of applying metalliferous wastes to land is bound up with management. Obviously there is no risk if small amounts of sludge such as 10 ton/hectare are applied, once for all, scattered over large areas, at least with normal soils. The risk involved in irrigating with treated effluent containing traces of heavy metals in solution is also very small, since again the amounts concerned are so small. The risk becomes serious when metalliferous sludge is applied repeatedly and in heavy amounts, so that zinc accumulates to a ton to the hectare or more, and other metals in corresponding amounts.

We have seen that crops have been grown successfully where the total application of zinc has been far above any commonly recommended figure. This practice may still be criticized for two reasons: one, that some leafy vegetables cannot be grown on that soil; the other, that the success even with the cereals is temporary, and that as the organic matter oxidizes away the metals will become progressively more toxic to all crops.

On the first score, one can arrange all plants in a list from the most sensitive to the most resistant. Since resistance to zinc (or to other heavy metals) has not yet been considered in breeding, one may confidently predict that resistant strains will be found or created throughout this list. But given that some plants will be ruled out, even with the best agricultural treatment, the practical question to be decided is whether these sensitive crops are grown over a large enough area to matter. This is not the place to debate a social decision, but it may be pointed out here that 70% of the cropped area of the United States grows the stock cereals and soybeans which are not sensitive to the common heavy metals, while the sensitive beets and leafy vegetables comprise 1.5%; the sensitivity of some other nongramineous crops is not known.

The second score concerns science rather than policy, and this calls for our attention here, namely to consider how far a suitable management may meet the above threat of toxicity to crops in general.

The two variable features of soil under control are organic content and pH. One other favorable feature of sewage wastes, namely high phosphate content, will persist for many years, and as discussed earlier it may help in immobilizing or antagonizing toxic metals. But the organic content and pH may change with time, and the organic content gives the greater cause for concern. Obviously there is a limit to the amount of zinc which can be inactivated by a ton of organic matter. Yet the zinc is in the soil once and for all, while the organic matter is open to microbial attack. So the question arises, How rapidly will the added organic matter be oxidized away?

At present this question cannot be answered with certainty. But some theories and experimental evidence will be discussed which should enable us to predict with good prospects of success. We may first discuss the problem in simple form, bearing in mind that some modifications will later be needed.

4.6.1 Organic Content and Management

For any climate, plant cover, and soil, there must eventually be a stable percentage of organic matter (O. M.), whether high or medium or low; this is obviously the figure which we find in a virgin soil. When this stable figure has been reached, then the addition of organic carbon in any one year by fixation of CO_2 (mostly by higher plants) equals the oxidation of organic carbon to CO_2 by respiration of microbes, plants, and animals. Generally we may analyze this as a balance between plants as builders and microbes as destroyers, and this will be the theme here, though in hot and dry climates at least we must invoke destruction by animals such as termites to help explain the low organic content.

The two main components of soil climate are water supply and temperature. Generally the wetter and cooler the situation the higher the organic content of the soil, since bacteria are more inhibited by poor aeration and cold than higher plants are. The steady state can be expressed by the equation $A = S \cdot r$, where A = annual addition of O. M. in tons per hectare, S = total amount of O. M. in tons per hectare, and r = proportion of this oxidized in a year. (Therefore, $S = A/r$.) The relation is a ratio. The unfortunate idea that it is a difference between amount added and amount destroyed is still widely repeated in books, though it implies not merely zero O. M. at high temperature, but even more absurd, a negative amount. Sometimes this absurdity is expressed in so many words: "Organic matter in the tropics decomposes more rapidly than it is formed."

This simple formula relates to totals; total carbon fixed equals total carbon released. The total comprises a wide range of A's, each with its own r, though it is useful to confine the discussion to the more stable A's, and to ignore the trash which will disappear within the year.

The ratio depends not only on water supply and temperature, but also on chemical fertility. In any one district one soil may be found with twice the organic content of another because it is rich in phosphate while the other is poor. In this case the plants are greatly helped by the phosphate; no doubt the bacteria are also helped, but not to such an extent.

In passing from the natural (or neolithic) state to industrial domination, two opposing things happen: (1) tops are harvested and removed and perhaps straw is burned; (2) fertilizer is added which increases roots and stubble or increases the leguminous crops which add nitrogen to the soil. For any one rotation or system of management a new equilibrium is reached where the O. M. may be more or less than in prehuman nature. Far too much has been made, and is being made, of the theme that inhuman nature is bountiful and that man has abused her bounty. True enough, it is common for pioneers to plunder any stored wealth, to fell and burn the forest and grow potatoes in the ashes. But the opposite is just as common, and in Australia it has been the rule; over millions of hectares superphosphate with or without trace elements has established leguminous plants and started the accumulation of O. M. on pasture land to unprecedented levels. Cropland shows the same effect; on naturally poor sandy farmland in Western Australia one can see where superphosphate has been added by the darker soil — more roots had grown where the phosphorus was added, besides the good crop above ground of which the grain had been harvested.

In longer settled land, one might quote here the Dutch work [96] with the record of more O. M. and better structure following practices where more roots had been left in the soil; cereal crops led to satisfactory O. M. content and good structure, while potatoes and beets led to much poorer structure. Obviously there is an appropriate A for each kind of management, and therefore an S to which it will converge.

But this analysis has so far made too little distinction among kinds of O. M., other than the note that one may omit the most transient kind from one's calculations. In order to introduce one most important distinction it is helpful first to consider three features of soil O. M. that are commonly listed in the books when its benefits are being set out.

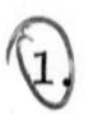

1. Physical features: It confers good structure by binding the very fine particles of clay and silt together into aggregates the size of sand. Thus the addition of O. M. makes soil softer, easier to work, and less beaten down and dispersed by rain.

2. Nutritional and biological features: It provides through microbial action for soluble nitrogen and sulfur to be released to plants at a steady rate, fast enough for all needs, but not in such excess as to be lost to drainage. Phosphorus may often be added to this list.

3. Chemical features: By virtue of its negative charge it holds a supply of cations in the exchangeable form. These cations include the nutrients Ca, Mg, K, Na, NH_4, Mn, and some other trace elements. There is a small analogy between this effect and the second, in that the exchangeable ions also may be slowly released to plants as needed, but in the second the organic molecule is destroyed, while here the organic base remains unchanged while the cations move in and out.

What must be emphasized here is that the second and third virtues are mutually exclusive. As soon as the humic molecule is attacked by microbes and its nitrogen converted to ammonium, it has disappeared as a protector against the metals. Or putting it the other way, if it is to be permanently useful in holding the metals, it must keep its nitrogen permanently locked up. That is, there are two different organic matters, temporary and permanent. German writers have used the words Nahrhumus (nahr = nourish) and Dauerhumus (dauer = endure), but their English equivalents are little used as yet. Even with the physical virtues the same distinction applies. Some soils high in O. M. have good structure which is due to their Dauerhumus. But many soils with modest levels of O. M. also have good structure, and farmers have long recognized the good and temporary effects of some green manures. One component that is so responsible is polyuronide, a linear molecule that ties other particles together; a product from both plants and microbes that is itself subject to microbial attack. This is effective at the rate of 200 kg/ha. A synthetic copy of it ("Krilium") was used in the field 20 years ago and had substantial practical success.

It is of course conceivable that a humic colloid could be simultaneously Nahr and Dauer, if every such molecule were to live for about 20 years and its place were taken, on its dissolution, by a freshly synthesized molecule. But this is certainly not so. There are two lines of evidence for this, one old and one new. The old line follows the observation that when good land is broken up its O. M. declines — rapidly for some years, but then much more slowly. It is the later almost constant lower level that concerns us here; eventually the Dauerhumus greatly predominates over the Nahrhumus. The new line is the measurement of C-14 in the soil; the older the O. M. the more of the active isotope will have decayed. The age of O. M. varies among soils, but a common figure for the average age is 500 years. The figure is comparible with many ratios of contemporary to old — of Nahrhumus to Dauerhumus — depending on the age of the old; it may well turn out that Nahrhumus makes up no more than one-fourth of the total.

But if the Dauerhumus is so old, it is decomposing only very slowly, and if, as we may reasonably suppose, it keeps at a steady value, it can receive only small increments annually. (Scharpenseel [97] suggests 20 kg/ha annually.) From these considerations, one should not expect to make a permanent addition even by adding much more O. M. than the soil originally held. One qualification may be made to this argument -- namely, that since the O. M. by forming a strong bond protects the roots from the zinc, we should also expect the zinc to protect the O. M. from the microbes. Campbell et al. [98] quote metallic humates having a greater age than humic acids; however, this concerns the stability of Dauerhumus already formed, not of hypothetical Dauerhumus in course of formation. Such measurements as we have at present of the rate of disappearance of O. M. when metalliferous sludge has been applied to the reclamation of wasteland do not support this hopeful argument -- it disappears at the regular rate.

One might also argue that the abundant phosphate of the sludged soil will favor a high organic content. But the prudent basis for calculations is that the organic content is destined to return to the normal value for that climate and that management, this word comprising not only choice between crops, but bare fallowing on one hand and grazing of pasture on the other.

The most detailed published study of the effect of added sludge on the organic content of soil is the work of Mann and Barnes [99], in which a sandy soil was cropped for 9 years with vegetables, treated annually with either farmyard manure, composts, or sludge, and analyzed regularly for organic nitrogen and carbon. The soil without these additions kept its O. M. constant at 1.6% (that is, income equalling oxidation). Adding 75 tons/ha each of farmyard manure and sludge annually, representing respectively a total of 103 tons and 154 tons of dry O. M. over the 9 years, they found that the additional O. M. in the soil represented 49% (for manure) and 55% (for sludge) of the amount added. From these figures one may compute the annual rate of oxidation to be close to 20% and 15%, respectively, using the following argument.

If the annual addition is A tons and the proportion annually oxidized is r, then the amount remaining after 9 years is

$$S = A\ [1 + (1-r) + (1-r)^2 + \ldots + (1-r)^8] = A/r\ [1 - (1-r)^9]$$

which leads to the above figures. This formula, by the way, leads eventually to the simple $S = A/r$ when the number of years is large.

One could match the experimental figures just as well by assuming that r is higher for the first year after application and lower for all subsequent years. But this device of dividing the manure or sludge into very active and very inert fractions cannot be carried far. If one assumes a regular annual loss less than 10% after the first year, the first year's loss must be made unreasonably high in order to balance the account. Without doubt many more figures will become available during the next few years, from which values for r may be computed. One experience should be mentioned here, namely at Ottawa, Illinois, where a heavy application of sludge was used to reclaim a waste alkaline sand, with grasses being successfully grown as described by Peterson et al. [85]. In a recent check it was found that 4 years after treatment the ratio of Cr to O. M. was close to twice that of the original sludge (after allowing for the small O. M. of the unimproved soil), corresponding to r between 0.15 and 0.20, since the Cr is itself a measure of how much sludge was added.

If we now suppose that good crops continue to be grown, so favoring a satisfactory equilibrium value for the O. M., we can see that if we make r = 0.15 it takes only 4 to 5 years for an application of 200 tons of added O.M. (as sludge) to decline to 100 tons. Thus if the receiving soil itself can inactivate heavy metals as well as does 100 tons of O.M. from fresh sludge, the burden of the heavy metals will have increased by 50% in 4 to 5 years and doubled in 8 or 9.

A further calculation here may show the order of figures in which we are dealing. The O.M. of soil has a cation exchange capacity of about 250 meq/100 g at pH 6 and 350 meq/100 g at pH 7. If all this were satisfied by zinc, this would mean 8% by weight at pH 6 and 11.2% at pH 7. If a tolerant crop such as corn remains healthy when O.M. is 5% saturated with zinc at pH 6 and 20% at pH 7, and that soil O.M. at equilibrium weighs 100 ton/hectare, then 0.4 ton Zn will be looked after by the O.M. at pH 6 and 2.2 tons at pH 7.

4.6.2 A New Case for Liming

Emphasis has been given in the preceding pages to the protective effect of the organic fraction. This has always attracted most attention since it is the first reason why sludge on its first application does nothing but good. Yet some observers might prefer to think of this first good effect as being only a temporary makeshift, and would advise that reliance should rather be placed on lime.

As pointed out in the introductory sections, raising the pH of soil increases the adsorption of heavy metals, and in the formula for safe limits in applying a metalliferous sludge it was suggested that additional allowance should be made for each increase of 0.5 pH. Thus advice about sludge is usually coupled with advice to add enough lime to keep soil pH above 6.5.

Now this is traditional farming advice. True, many commercial crops do not need such a high pH, and a few can be damaged by it. But for most crops it is good advice and in simple chemical terms it can be described as a method of keeping the noxious elements Al and Mn out of the way. We now have an additional reason

— to keep Zn and Ni and Cd out of the way. It is a difference of detail, not of principle.

Most reports on the heavy metals are in keeping with this advice, and perhaps the most important is the finding that the uptake of Cd is less at higher pH. At the same time, the situation is not one of simple routine. High uptakes of both Zn [80] and Ni [8] have been reported at high pH, though damage to crops was then reduced. The most substantial published experiment showing damage with zinc used conditions remote from the field [57], with a heavy application of $Zn(NO_3)_2$ unaccompanied by leaching.

4.6.3 The Effect of Poor Drainage

Almost all the economic crops require good drainage, rice being the best known exception. It has been assumed in all the foregoing discussion that drainage is normal. The question arises whether the impact of heavy metals in a soil is made more severe by poor drainage.

Manganese can be liberated from MnO_2 by waterlogging — that is, by anaerobic conditions; and there are records of toxic Mn being thus produced and damaging orchards. However, this piece of chemistry is peculiar to manganese, and we are concerned here with zinc and its associates in sludge.

At present little information is available. There is little reason to expect the cations (other than Mn^{2+}) to be so liberated, though, of course, a heavy metal that was trapped within MnO_2 would be liberated if the crystal were broken up. But possibly a greater amount of chelated heavy metal might circulate, as new organic molecules are formed in the waterlogged soil; it is difficult to see how this could create any worse conditions than there were when the original sludge, with its own anaerobic history, was mixed in.

Two pieces of work come to mind here. One is the study by Ng and Bloomfield [100] of the liberation of trace elements from soils that were waterlogged with fermenting grasses. (But this concerns the attack of bacterial products on mineral silicates rather than on already chelated zinc.) The other is the pedological evidence of Mitchell [31] that more heavy metals are extractable from poorly drained than from well-drained soils. Whether this would be true of sludged soils is not known.

4.6.4 Harvesting the Foreign Metal

Some of the high figures quoted for heavy metals in plants raise the thought that the unwanted accumulation of a foreign metal might be harvested by growing a specialist crop, just as we harvest N, sometimes to the extent of impoverishing a soil. This does not seem likely for the elements here concerned when sludge is applied heavily. (For example, a crop of 10 tons containing the high amount of 500 ppm Zn removes only 5 kg from a hectare.) The most promising such suggestion has been made for Mo, which has an unusually wide range of concentrations in plants, from below 0.1 to 100 ppm. Thus a 5-ton crop of a specialist collector would remove 500 g from a hectare; the fiber crop ramie is said to be such a specialist. This might be significant for some agricultural purpose where the available Mo was only 5 kg/ha and grazing stock were afflicted with molybdenosis. But for annual light applications, as with irrigation, the above removal of 5 kg Zn would balance the income from effluent of 100 cm annually containing 0.5 mg/liter Zn.

4.6.5 A Possible Day of Reckoning

The preceding pages have dealt with the problem of living with additional heavy metals in the soil; let us speak here of zinc, since it is the most active of the foreign metals, and present in highest amounts in sludge if not in effluent. We have discussed how the zinc may be held harmless over years of periodic addition. Normally a manager would cease adding metalliferous waste long before the situation became critical. But we may suppose that the organic matter is no longer sufficient to hold the Zn, that the land can no longer grow the preferred crops, and that only a few specially tolerant crops may now be grown. We may briefly consider the possibility of removing the zinc-laden topsoil and starting afresh with the subsurface. True, there is a popular prejudice that subsoil is permanently bad; but this is irrational. The fault of poor structure may be cured by adding O.M., both from outside and through growing plants in the new surface; and any chemical deficiencies may be made good. Since the previous history of this new soil has involved the addition of much N and P and O.M. above it, it will have benefited from that more than any ordinary subsoil. So our chemical problem is to estimate how far the new soil starts with a handicap on account of foreign metals. From the foregoing pages, it seems likely that its load of Ni, Pb, and Cd will be low. Its load of Zn may not be high, though by the time that the Zn has become mobile enough to limit the growth of all but the most tolerant plants it must have accumulated somewhat in the second 15 cm as well as the first. For the Cu it is more difficult to say; perhaps Cu in organic combination will have moved downwards also, but from all that we know here a dangerous excess is most unlikely. An alternative to removing the top few centimeters would be to bury to 1 meter deep by complete inversion. But it is not our purpose here to discuss the feasibility in economic terms, only to comment on the chemistry.

CHAPTER 5

TWO FUTURE INQUIRIES

5.1 PRACTICE AND THEORY

It has been common in man's use of soils that practice has run ahead of theory, and our present topic is no exception. The early work on trace elements, when we learned which of them were essential and recognized their deficiency in the field, did not derive from soil studies. The opposite happened — such theories as were developed came after the field work. So too today, when we want to know how much of a foreign metal may safely be applied to a soil, we are hastening to test the performance of various plants on soils to which various burdens of metals have been added at various levels of pH and organic matter, and any new theory will come later.

As may have occurred to the reader of the preceding pages, there are two lines of inquiry on which more theoretical understanding would help practical progress, dealing with soils and plants, respectively.

On soils, our ideas on what is here called "reversion" are vague. There is a current view that is somewhat akin to laissez-faire in economics; namely, that if one leaves the system alone, it will come out right eventually. This view has merit when dealing with small amounts, but when we deal with hundreds of kilograms per hectare we must learn about the actual forms in which Zn and the others are held before we assume that they are on their way to burial, like the B in tourmaline, which can never become toxic, or the P and Mo buried in ferric oxides, which can never become nutritious.

First, organic matter cannot account for reversion to forgettable forms of a heavy metal. Not only is its capacity limited, and the competition for a place severe, but it does not recrystallize so does not become less soluble with time — rather the opposite, as we have just discussed. So, if the heavy metal is to be buried, it must be in an inorganic form. It is clear that soils do not contain a universal mechanism for such a disposal, as shown by the toxicity of soils developed on serpentine — on silicate, that is. The suggestion is given here (Section 2.3.7) that Fe_2O_3 is not a promising burial ground and that MnO_2 is much more promising (Section 2.6.1); but in practice soils containing even as much as 200 ppm of Mn as active MnO_2 are rare.

A theoretical reliance on the high specific surface of soils calls for the following calculation. If we accept the physical chemists' conclusions that ions adsorbed on a surface cannot be denser than one charge to 20 square angstroms (2,000 nm^2), this amounts to an upper limit of 1 meq/100 g siliceous material of diameter 0.002 mm (a negligible figure), and of 10 meq/100 g of diameter 0.0002 mm. It would involve 10% saturation with the heavy metals against competitors to account thus for a <u>surface</u> (not a <u>reverted</u>) holding of 300 ppm.

The above reasoning leads to the second line of inquiry, which assumes that mankind, while taking due precautions against Cd, must learn to live with the other heavy metals in soils, as he lives with acidic or saline or calcareous soils, by choosing or even breeding his crops. Our program of selection would be helped if we had more fundamental knowledge of how plants deal with each foreign metal and how it damages them. This involves comparison of our common plants with those that have evolved to carry high concentrations of unusual elements without damage. This is one example of a general principle, that the study of life in unusual environments can throw light on life in normal environments.

REFERENCES

1. Aung Khin and G. W. Leeper, Agrochim., 4:246-254 (1960).
2. C. H. Williams and J. R. Simpson, Aust. J. Agric. Res., 16:412-427 (1965).
3. For a nonspecialist summary see L. Pokras, J. Chem. Educ., 33:152, 223, 283 (1950).
4. E. J. Russell and J. A. Prescott, J. Agric. Sci., 8:65-110 (1916).
5. K. G. Tiller, Trans. 9th Internat. Cong. Soil Sci., II:567-575.
6. R. D. Johnson, R. L. Jones, T. D. Hinesly, and D. J. David, Selected Chemical Characteristics of Soils, Forages, and Drainage Waters from the Sewage Farm Serving Melbourne, Australia. Prepared for Corps of Engineers, U.S.A., 1974 (typescript).
7. F. Steenbjerg, Tids. Planteavl, 39:401-441 (1933).
8. M. M. Crooke, Soil Sci., 81:269-276 (1956).
9. L. H. P. Jones, S. C. Jarvis, and D. W. Cowling, Plant and Soil, 38:605-619 (1973).
10. R. O. James and T. W. Healy, J. Coll. Interf. Sci., 40:42-81 (1972).
11. F. Vydra and J. Galba, Coll. Czech. Chem. Commun., 34:3471-3478 (1969).

12. Notably E. A. Jenne in "Trace Inorganics in Water", Adv. Chem. Ser., 73 (1968).

13a. H. van Dijk, Geoderma, 5:53-67 (1961).

13b. J. B. Passioura and G. W. Leeper, Agrochim., 8:81-90 (1963).

14. F. L. Himes and S. A. Barber, Soil Sci. Soc. Amer. Proc., 21:368-373 (1957).

15. D. S. Gamble and M. Schnitzer, The Chemistry of Fulvic Acid and its Reactions with Metal Ions, in P. C. Singer (ed.), "Trace Metals and Metal-Organic Interactions in Natural Waters," pp. 265-302, Ann Arbor Sci., Ann Arbor, Michigan, 1973.

16. J. F. Hodgson, H. R. Geering, and W. A. Norvell, Soil Sci. Soc. Amer. Proc., 29:665-669 (1965).

17. J. F. Hodgson, W. L. Lindsay, and J. F. Trierweiler, Soil Sci. Soc. Amer. Proc., 30:723-726 (1966).

18. H. R. Geering and J. F. Hodgson, Soil Sci. Soc. Amer. Proc., 33:54-59 (1969).

19. K. Norrish, Trans. 9th Internat. Cong. Soil Sci., II:713-723 (1968).

20. G. W. Leeper, "Six Trace Elements in Soils," pp. 37-40, Melbourne University Press, Melbourne, 1970.

21. R. L. Follett and W. L. Lindsay, Soil Sci. Soc. Amer. Proc., 35:600-602 (1971).

22. C. H. Williams and D. J. David, Aust. J. Soil Res., 11:43-56 (1973).

23. A. Heydemann, Geochim. Cosmochim. Acta, 15:305-329 (1959).

24. J. Muller, Ann. Agron., 11:75-91 (1960).

25. J. Delas, Agrochim., 7:258-288 (1963).

26. W. Reuther and P. W. Smith, Proc. Soil Sci. Soc. Florida, 14:17-23 (1954).

27. E. Steeman Nielsen and S. Wium-Andersen, Marine Biol., 6:93-97 (1970).

28. A. Siegel, Metal-Organic Interactions in the Marine Environment, in S. D. Faust and J. V. Hunter (eds.), "Organic Compounds in Aquatic Environments," pp. 265-295, Dekker, New York, 1971.

29. J. A. Roth, E. F. Wallihan, and R. G. Sharpless, Soil Sci., 112:338-342 (1971).

30. J. R. Kline and R. H. Rust, Soil Sci. Soc. Amer. Proc., 30: 188-192 (1966).

31. R. L. Mitchell, in Trace Elements in Soils, in F. E. Bear (ed.), "Chemistry of the Soil," 2d ed., American Chemical Society, Washington, D.C., 1964.

32. W. H. Durum and J. D. Hem, H. C. Hopps and H. L. Cannon (eds.), in "Geochemical Environment in Relation to Health and Disease," Annals of the New York Academy of Science, New York, 1972.

33. H. V. Warren, Endeavour, 31:46-49 (1972).

34. H. W. van der Marel, Soil Sci., 64:445-451 (1947).

35. J. Webber, Water Pollution Control, 71:404-412 (1972).

36. J. Lounamaa, Ann. Bot. Soc. "Vanamo," 29:4 (1956).

37. H. H. LeRiche and A. H. Weir, J. Soil Sci., 14:225-235 (1963).

38. R. M. McKenzie, Aust. J. Soil Res., 5:235-246 (1967).

39. K. D. Nicolls and J. L. Honeysett, Aust. J. Agric. Res., 15: 368-376 (1964).

40. K. D. Nicolls and J. L. Honeysett, Aust. J. Agric. Res., 15: 609-624 (1964).

41. R. M. McKenzie, Aust. J. Soil Res., 8:97-106 (1970).

42. See for example J. R. Wright, R. Levick, and H. J. Atkinson, Soil Sci. Soc. Amer. Proc., 19:340-344 (1955).

43. J. Morgan, Adv. Chem. Ser., 67:1-29 (1967).

44. L. H. P. Jones and K. A. Handreck, Adv. Agron., 19:107-149 (1967).

45. J. C. Moonaw, M. T. Nakamura, and G. D. Sherman, Pacific Sci., 13:335-341 (1959).

46. R. P. G. Gregory and A. D. Bradshaw, New Phytol., 64:131-143 (1965).

47. The subject of tolerance is reviewed by J. Antonovics, A. D. Bradshaw, and R. G. Turner, Adv. Ecol. Res., 7:1-85 (1971).

48. W. R. Dykeman and A. S. de Sousa, Can. J. Bot., 44:871-878 (1966).

49. K. A. Smith, Plant and Soil, 34:369-379 (1971).

50. J. C. Brown and W. D. Bell, Soil Sci. Soc. Amer. Proc., 33:99-101 (1969).

51. J. C. Brown, J. E. Ambler, R. L. Chaney, and C. D. Foy, in J. J. Mortvedt, P. M. Giordano, and W. L. Lindsay (eds.), "Micronutrients in Agriculture," Soil Science Society of America, Madison, Wisconsin, 1972.

52. O. W. Nicolls, D. M. J. Provan, M. M. Cole, and J. S. Tooms, Trans. Inst. Min. Met., 74:695-799 (1965).

53. M. D. Carroll and J. F. Loneragan, Aust. J. Agric. Res., 19:859-868 (1968).

54. J. Vlamis and D. E. Williams, Plant and Soil, 27:131-140 (1967).

55. J. E. Bowen, Plant and Soil, 37:577-588 (1972).

56. S. C. Jarvis, L. H. P. Jones, and M. J. Hopper, Plant and Soil, 44:179-191 (1976).

57. L. C. Boawn and P. E. Rasmussen, Agron. J., 63:874-876 (1971).

58. L. C. Boawn, Soil Sci. Plant Anal., 2(1):31-36 (1971).

59. E. J. Underwood, "Trace Elements in Human and Animal Nutrition", 3d ed., p. 269, Academic Press, New York, 1971.

60. L. M. Walsh, W. H. Erhardt, and H. D. Siebel, J. Environ. Quality, 1:197-200 (1972).

61. C. F. Mills and A. C. Dalgarno, Nature, 239:171-173 (1972).

62. L. Friberg, "Cadmium in the Environment," Academic Press, New York, 1974.

63. A. L. Page, F. T. Bingham, and C. Nelson, J. Environ. Qual., 1:288-291 (1972).

64. J. Webber, "Cadmium in the Environment," pp. 13-14, Inter-Research Council Committee on Pollution Research, London, 1973.

65. A. J. Anderson, D. R. Meyer, and F. K. Mayer, Aust. J. Agric. Res., 24:557-571 (1973).

66. R. L. Halstead, Can. J. Soil. Sci., 48:301-305 (1968).

67. R. L. Halstead, B. J. Finn, and A. J. McLean, Can. J. Soil Sci., 49:335-342 (1969).

68. L. H. P. Jones, C. R. Clement, and M. J. Hopper, Plant and Soil, 38:403-414 (1973).

69. A. J. McLean, R. L. Halstead, and B. J. Finn, Can. J. Soil Sci., 49:327-334 (1969).

70. M. L. Berrow and J. Webber, J. Sci. Fd. Agric., 23:93-100 (1972).

71. R. B. Dean and J. E. Smith, The Properties of Sludges, in "Recycling Municipal Sludges and Effluents on Land", pp. 39-47, National Association of State Universities and Land-Grant Colleges, Washington D.C., 1973.

72. A. J. Kaplovsky and E. Genetelli, "Land Disposal of Municipal Effluents and Sludges," p. 11 (U.S. EPA-902/9-73-001), Rutgers University, New Jersey 1973.

73. L. A. Klein, M. Lang, N. Nash, and S. L. Kirschner, J. Water Poll. Control Fed., 46:2653-2662 (1974).

74. J. R. Peterson, C. Lue-Hing, and D. R. Zenz, "Recycling Treated Municipal Wastewater and Sludge through Forest and Cropland," pp. 26-37, Pennsylvania State University Press, 1973.

75. F. Steenbjerg and E. Boken, Plant and Soil, 2:195-221 (1950).

76. S. H. Jenkins and J. S. Cooper, Inter. J. Air Water Poll., 8: 695-703 (1964).

77. L. D. King and H. D. Morris, J. Environ. Qual., 1:425-429 (1972).

78. J. R. Peterson and J. Gschwind, J. Environ. Qual., 1:410-412 (1972).

79. J. B. E. Patterson, Min. Ag. Fish. Food Tech. Bull., 21: HMSO, London, 1971.

80. R. L. Chaney, Crop and Food Chain Effects of Toxic Elements in Sludges and Effluents, in "Recycling Municipal Sludges and Effluents on Land", pp. 129-141, National Association of State Universities and Land-Grant Colleges, Washington, D.C., 1973.

81. G. Rohde, Wasserwirts. Wassertech. (WWT), 11:542-550 (1961).

82. G. Rohde, J. Inst. Sew. Purif., 581-585 (1962).

83. S. Trocmé, G. Barbier, and J. Chabannes, Ann. Agron., 1: 663-685 (1950).

84. T. D. Hinesly, R. L. Jones, and E. L. Ziegler, Compost Sci., 26-30 (1972).

85. J. R. Peterson, T. M. McCalla, and G. E. Smith, in R. A. Olson (ed.), "Fertilizer Technology and Use," 2d ed., Soil Science Society of America, 1971.

86. C. Lue-Hing, B. T. Lyman, J. R. Peterson, and J. G. Gshwind, Chicago Prairie Plan - A Report on Eight Years of Municipal Sewage Sludge Utilization, in R. C. Loehr (ed.), "Land as a Waste Management Alternative," pp. 551-581, Ann Arbor Sci., Ann Arbor, 1977.

87. C. G. Chumbley, A. D. A. S. Advisory Paper No. 10, Min. Agric. Fisheries and Food, 1971.

88. Discussed in "Factors Involved in Land Application of Agricultural and Municipal Wastes," Agricultural Research Service, United States Department of Agriculture, Beltsville, Maryland, 1974.

89. D. E. Baker and L. Chesnin, Adv. Agron., 27:305-374 (1975).

90. For collections of American figures on effluents see this and the following reference: A. Z. Mytelka, J. S. Czachor,

W. B. Gaggino, and H. Golub, J. Water Poll. Control Fed., 45:1859-1864 (1973).

91. P. A. Blakeslee, Monitoring Considerations for Municipal Wastewater Effluent and Sludge Application to the Land, in "Recycling Municipal Sludges and Effluents on Land", pp. 183-198, National Association of State Universities and Land-Grant Colleges, Washington D.C., 1973.

92. H. V. Warren, R. E. Delavault, and K. W. Fletcher, Can. Min. Met. Bull., 64:34-45 (July 1971).

93. D. Purves, Trans. 9th Internat. Cong. Soil Sci., II:351-355 (1968).

94. L. Linnman, A. Andersson, K. O. Nilsson, B. Lind, T. Kjellstrom, and L. Friberg, Arch. Environ. Health, 27:45-47 (1973).

95. A. Andersson and K. P. Nilsson, Ambio, 3:99-101 (1974).

96. P. K. Peerlkamp, 4th Internat. Cong. Soil Sci., I:50-54 (1950).

97. H. W. Scharpenseel, Special Methods of Chromatographic and Radiometric Analysis, in A. D. McLaren and J. Skujins (eds.), "Soil Biochemistry" Vol. 2, pp. 96-128, Dekker, New York, 1971.

98. C. A. Campbell, E. A. Paul, D. A. Rennie, and K. J. McCallum, Soil Sci., 104:217-224 (1967).

99. H. H. Mann and T. W. Barnes, J. Agric. Sci., 48:160-163 (1957).

100. Ng, Siew Kee and C. Bloomfield, Plant and Soil, 16:108-135 (1962).

REVIEWS AND SOURCES

Reviews and symposia are fashionable in every field. This book has the aim of summarizing the present state of knowledge, not of being bibliographic. Many books and articles are available with long lists of published articles; some of these are comprehensive, others are selective, sometimes both kinds being represented within one publication. The following list contains bibliographic material as well as reviews. It is intended for any reader who wishes more detailed information on our subject, so differing in intention from the accompanying list of references quoting the authority for particular statements.

Allaway, W. H., Environmental Cycling of Trace Elements, Adv. Agron., 20:235-271 (1968).

Chaney, R. L., S. B. Hornick, and P. W. Simon, Heavy Metal Relationships during Land Utilization of Sewage Sludge in the Northeast, in R. C. Loehr (ed.), "Land as a Waste Management Alternative", pp. 283-314 (Ann Arbor Sci., Ann Arbor, 1977). (A review of many long-term farming experiences, with much attention to cadmium.)

Chapman, H. D., (ed.), "Diagnostic Criteria for Plants and Soils," University of California, Berkeley, 1966. (Mostly concerned with deficiency.)

Hopps, H. C., and H. L. Cannon (eds.), "Geochemical Environment in Relation to Health and Disease," Annals New York Academy of Science, 199 (1972).

Leeper, G. W., "Six Trace Elements in Soils", Melbourne University Press, Melbourne, 1970.

Lisk, D. J., Trace Metals in Soils, Plants, and Animals, Adv. Agron. 24:267-311 (1972). (With tables of contents of many metals in soil, water, plant, and animal.)

Mitchell, R. L., Trace Elements in Soils, in F. E. Bear (ed.), "Chemistry of the Soil", 2nd ed., American Chemical Society Monograph, 1964.

Mortvedt, J. J., P. M. Giordano, and W. L. Lindsay (eds.), "Micronutrients in Agriculture," Soil Science Society of America, Madison, Wisconsin, 1972.

Page, A. L., "Fate and Effects of Trace Elements in Sewage Sludge when Applied to Agricultural Lands, a Literature Review Study," U.S. Environmental Protection Agency, National Environmental Health Center, Cincinnati, Ohio, 1974.

Swaine, D. J., "Trace Elements in Soils," Commonwealth Bureau of Soils Tech. Comm. 48, Commonwealth Bureau of Soils, Harpenden, Herts, England, 1955. (Statistical summary.)

Warren, H. V., Biogeochemistry in Canada, Endeavour, 31:46-49 (1972).

Cadmium has received special attention in recent years. The following three recent reviews, with special regard to health, may be consulted.

Fulkerson, W., and H. E. Goeller (eds.), "Cadmium the Dissipated Element," Oak Ridge National Laboratory, Oak Ridge, Tennessee, TS, 513 pp., Jan. 1973.

Friberg, L., "Cadmium in the Environment," Academic Press, New York, 1974.

Environmental Health Perspectives for May 1974, experimental issue no. 7, pp. 253-323, U.S.A. Government Printing Office, Washington, D.C., 1974.

INDEX OF SYSTEMATIC NAMES

SYSTEMATIC NAMES OF PLANTS REFERRED TO IN BOOK

Common name	Systematic name
barley	Hordeum vulgare
barley grass (Werribee farm)	Hordeum leporinum
beet	Beta vulgaris
black spruce	Picea mariana
brazil nut	Bertholletia excelsa
cabbage	Brassica oleracea
calamine violet	Viola calaminaria
celery	Apium graveolens
colonial bentgrass	Agrostis tenuis
corn (U.S. usage)	Zea mays
docks	Rumex spp.
hydrangea	Hydrangea macrophylla
larch	Larix laricina
leeks	Allium porrum
lettuce	Lactuca sativa
maize	Zea mays
oats	Avena sativa
pineapple	Ananas comosus
potato	Solanum tuberosum

Common name	Systematic name
radish	Raphanus sativus
ramie	Boehmeria nivea
ryegrass	Lolium perenne
snapbean	Phaseolus vulgaris
soybean	Glycine max
spinach	Spinacea oleracea
subterranean clover	Trifolium subterraneum
sudan grass	Sorgum vulgare
sweetcorn	Zea mays
Swiss chard	Beta vulgaris
water couch	Paspalum distichum
wheat	Triticum aestivum

INDEX

Acetic acid as extractant, 33, 38, 43, 53, 68
Adsorption of cations, 7, 13, 18, 24, 31, 88
affected by pH, 18
Aluminum, viii, 11, 46
Ammonium acetate as reagent, 17, 30, 33, 92
Amorphous forms, 12
Anionic forms, 10, 23, 26, 32, 35
Antagonism, 24
in animals, 35, 49, 56
in plants, 28, 48, 57, 71
Arcola, 80
Available element, estimates, 35

Barium, ix, 17, 34, 47
Beets, 51, 69
Berlin, 74
Biogeochemistry, 46
Biophilic distribution, 33

Cadmium, xvi, 28, 30, 37, 40, 41, 51, 54-59, 62-67, 80-82, 86, 90, 92
Cation exchange, 14
capacity, 14, 17, 21, 25, 53, 88, 100
of sludge, 68
Chelates:
soluble, 11, 23, 51, 101
insoluble, 22
Chelating reagent, 22, 30, 38, 51, 57
Chlorosis, 47, 74, 84
Chromium, 10, 13, 18, 26, 99
Coal ash, 29, 91
Cobalt, 8, 9, 13, 18, 34, 40, 42, 43
Colloids of soils, 7, 13
Copper, 19, 22, 24, 28, 31-33, 40, 47, 54, 71, 77, 90, 103
anionic, 22, 23, 25, 32, 51
Corn, 74, 80-85
Crandallite, 24

Dauerhumus, 97
Drainage, poor, 43, 101

Exchangeable, range of meaning, 17, 34

Ferric oxide as absorbent, 13, 24, 42, 88, 106
First-class supply, 6
"Foreign" metals, 3

Genetic difference in absorption, 9, 46, 47, 94
Goethite, 24
Gorceixite, 24

Harvesting elements, 12, 102
Heavy metals:
  anionic, 10
  availability, 35
  content in drainage, 25, 78, 82
  content in plants, 29, 35, 39, 40, 41, 47, 91-93
  content in soils, 40
  harvesting, 12, 102
  in effluent, xviii, 90
  listed, x, 2
  proposed limits to use, xv, 37, 86-88, 90
  reactions with sludge and soil, 11
  special chemistry, 10
  state in sludge, 67
Hydrolysis, 11, 18, 29, 33

Iron, viii, 13, 26, 47
  anionic, 51
Irrigation, 90
Itai itai, 56

Lead, xi, 17, 33, 40, 60, 92
Liming, 8, 27, 33, 59, 74, 82, 100
Luxury consumption, 35

Management, xiv, 93
Manganese, ix, 8, 22, 27, 36, 38, 40, 49, 71, 101
  dioxide as absorbent, 42, 88, 101, 106
Melbourne sewage farm, 16, 74
Mercury, xi, 34, 45, 82
Metastable state, 12, 46
Mineralized country, 47, 48
MOH ion, 18, 31
Molybdenum, xi, 8, 35, 42, 47, 102

Nahrhumus, 97
Nickel, 17, 22, 28, 33, 40, 49, 59, 69, 101
Nitrogen in sludge, xvii, 62, 65, 66, 85, 89

Organic colloid, 21, 32
  content of sludge, 66
  matter of soil, 95-100
Oxidation, 21, 27, 43, 99

Paris, 71
Peaty soils, 32, 47, 54, 59
Padology, 41, 102
pH and heavy metals, xii, 8, 17, 83, 88, 101
  changes in, 20, 88, 94
Phosphorus, xii, 5, 8, 9, 13, 23, 66, 88

Plumbogummites, 24
Pot tests, 45, 51
Profile, 43

Reduction, 21, 26, 39, 42
Reversion, 6, 87, 89, 91, 105

Second-class supply, 6, 9, 17
Seed, movement into, 48, 60, 80, 83
Selenium, 2, 47
Serpentine, 26, 49, 59, 106
Sewage farms, 70-79
Silicic acid, 5, 46, 50
Sludge composition and nature, 61
  proposed limits to use, 86
  results in agriculture, 68-70, 79-86
Soil extractants, 22, 36-39, 71, 76
Solution culture, 49, 54, 57
Soybeans, 47, 82, 93
Species difference in absorption, 9, 35, 94, 106
Stoichiometric forms, 12
Subsoil, 25, 103
Sulfide, 11, 21, 26, 66, 67
Swiss chard, 53
Synergism, 70

Temperature and uptake of heavy metals, 36
Thermodynamics, 12, 43
Third-class supply, 6, 9
Tin, 34
Titanium, 34
Total amount of element, 10

Waterlogging, 28, 72, 101

Zinc, xii, 8, 15, 20, 22, 23, 28, 29, 30, 37, 40, 50, 52, 53, 69, 71, 76, 77, 78, 80, 85, 90, 94, 100, 102
  "equivalent", 86